Aging Fitfully

Preserving Functional Fitness
Regardless of Age or Limitation

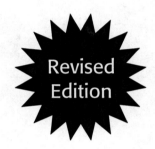

Revised
Edition

Sherrie Evenson, MS

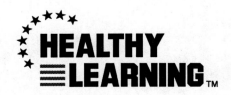

**HEALTHY
LEARNING**™

This book is intended to provide exercise guidance and information based on current knowledge in the scientific literature. Every effort has been made to ensure the information is accurate and up to date at the time of publication. It is expected that information will change over time and may modify information contained within this book.

Following the guidelines in this book is in no way intended to replace medical care, but to provide general principles. Consult your physician or other health professional for additional advice. Results are not guaranteed and will vary. The author is not responsible for injury resulting from any advice found in this book.

ISBN: 978-1-60679-063-2
Library of Congress Control Number: 2009924267
Cover design: Bean Creek Studio
Book layout: Bean Creek Studio
Front cover photo: ©2009 Jupiter Images Corporation
Back cover photo (top): ©2009 Jupiter Images Corporation
Back cover photo (bottom): Eric Griswold, Portland (OR)

Healthy Learning
P.O. Box 1828
Monterey, CA 93942
www.healthylearning.com

To Anna Duncan, my previous patient, dear friend, and inspiration. You are the ultimate example of "If she can do it, so can I."

Dedication

Acknowledgments

Many people reviewed this work for me, offered suggestions, gave positive feedback, and constructive criticism (i.e., "this woman is wordy"). I am grateful to these willing and honest professionals, clients, patients, family, and friends who took their valuable time to offer their observations and suggestions: Gary Ballew; Joann Bonneville, RN, BSN, Cardiopulmonary Rehabilitation; Mindy Baker, Fitness Technician, Wellness Assistant, Cherry Wood Village; Deborah K. Davis, DC; Mary Dedrick, MS, University of Buffalo, Buffalo, NY; Jim D. Duncan, Producer, Senior Showcase, Multnomah County Television (MCTV); Sandi Dykes, RN, FACVPR (Fellow, American Association of Cardiovascular and Pulmonary Rehabilitation); Malcolm Epley, Jr.; Janet Gonrowski, Marketing Communications Specialist; Jim Harding; Dennis Ludby; Jill Myers; Kristen Nelson; Paul Raukman; Frieda Reichsman, PhD, University of Massachusetts at Amherst; Judy Rice, RN, BA, Cardiopulmonary Rehabilitation; Erin Rose, BA, MPT, Wellness Center Director, Cherry Wood Village; Olivia Rossi, RN, MSN, ACSM Exercise Specialist®; Cheryl Schaffner, RN, MSN, Cardiopulmonary Rehabilitation; Chryss Toussaint, RN, BSN, OCN (Oncology Certified Nurse); and Mary Wilder, MD, Associate Professor, Western Seminary. Many thanks to technical writer Karen Demsey for her objective and professional editing expertise.

Thank you to my daughter, Kayla, for patience and understanding (at times reluctantly) when I had to say, "I'm sorry, I can't. I'm working on the book." And to Mom: I appreciate you allowing me to tell your story. It sets the perfect tone for the entire book, and speaks to the experience of many. I am proud to have you helping me with my mission.

Of course, those people are the obvious supporters. I don't want to forget the readers. Many thanks to those of you "out there" (and I hope you are many) who believe that this book can help you age fitfully. May it be so.

In memory of Tami

Contents

"All parts of the body which have a function, if used in moderation and exercised in labours in which each is accustomed, become thereby healthy, well-developed and age more slowly. But if unused and left idle, they become liable to disease, defective in growth, and age quickly."

—Hippocrates, Greek physician, 5th century, B.C

I have been pacing, impatient to cool down after my run. I am eager to get back to my book—your book. I am finally able to sit down, though still damp and overly warm.

Why so impatient? The fact that I was inspired to write this preface while out on my run is my first point. It's not uncommon for my greatest creativity to come to me when I am in motion. This attribute is not unique to me. Many people have been surprised and delighted by this somewhat underrated benefit of exercise, but in my view, one of the best.

The second reason I was moved to write this preface is that the run almost didn't happen. It had been a typical "book day." I had spent many hours at my easel, drawing many dozens of bodies demonstrating different exercises. My office was scattered with illustrations, open books, art pens, and erasers (used often). My only activity was to occasionally stand in front of my cheval mirror, placed in the doorway of my office, to strike a pose when I got confused about how an exercise should look. Should my knee show at that angle? What should my thumb be doing when I'm holding the band like this? Would this exercise be best drawn from the side or from the front?

This process went on for many hours. It was time to go run, but I was tired, stiff, and stressed. Though I knew exercise would help with each of these issues, sitting in the lounge chair outside on the deck with my feet up sounded ever so much better than pulling together the energy for a run. Does this surprise you? If you think that avid exercisers, even those who are exercise professionals, never struggle with motivation, you may be pleasantly surprised. I have exercised consistently since 1980, have been an exercise physiologist since 1982, and a competitive triathlete since I was in my 20s. Yet, sometimes getting out the door is the hardest part.

I have the benefit of many years of learning to override that voice that occasionally tries to lead me down the path of inactivity, and also the helpful obligation that I am a professional and have to be a good role model. Ironically, I think sometimes sharing my experience of "I don't wanna"—but doing it anyway—is the most professional, and helpful, thing to say. Playing the "purist" isn't necessarily motivating to others.

Motivation and time are two of the primary struggles in establishing a consistent exercise program. Clearly, I am not beyond an occasional loss of motivation. Further, with a very busy life, I can also relate to the time issue. Like many people, I'm routinely challenged to find time to squeeze in my exercise—sometimes even just that minimum 30 minutes.

Add a medical condition, injury, or chronic disease to the mix, and the ability to successfully exercise is even more challenging. Anything that makes it harder, or more painful, to move decreases the chances that one will be compliant with exercise. It can be hard enough when you are strong, healthy, and able.

I like to remember and remind people of the 20-80 principle: it's what you do 80 percent of the time that matters. The 20 percent is not what makes the notable difference. This principle hopefully helps to constructively deal with relapses, as success is really determined by how you handle life's interferences. When you have a temporary setback, do you get back on track, or do you experience "relapse collapse"?

I saw a quote on a refrigerator once that immediately struck me as utterly true:

"Unsuccessful people trade what they most want
for what they want in the moment."

I don't know who said this, but this simple wisdom has since revealed itself applied to many situations and circumstances. Today was one small example of how easy it would have been to indulge in "what I wanted in the moment." I could have easily rationalized how much I deserved some relaxation after working so hard, and sunk into the lounge chair (and that has happened). The danger is that "small examples," though seemingly insignificant in each isolated instance, can establish long-term patterns. Fortunately for me (this time anyway), I was able to override temptation, and was rewarded with an invigorating run. The stiffness, fatigue, and stress had vanished.

One thing we know about physical inactivity: it leads to more inactivity. The less you move, the less you want to move. You say you will start exercising when you get more energy? You need to start exercising. Energy will follow.

Fortunately, the converse is also true: physical activity leads to more activity. The more active you are, the easier it is to remain active. Not that you won't have those days that you just "don't wanna." And you will have days when *not* exercising will be a good idea. Exercise isn't always the healthy choice.

Just remember: it is what you choose to do 80 percent of the time that will make the difference.

Now, give yourself a gift. Arise. Go forth. Age fitfully.

STOP. PLEASE READ THIS PAGE.

THREE SECTIONS

This book is organized into three sections, Part One: Talking About It, Part Two: Doing It, and Appendix: Here to Help (Tools and References).

Part One: Talking About It provides a solid educational foundation, intended to help individuals, as well as those assisting others with their exercise program. It discusses the areas of aerobic fitness, muscular strength/endurance, flexibility, and balance. Current guidelines are addressed for healthy people as well as older individuals and people with disabilities. Included is a wealth of information for people who may deal with any number of health issues. Dozens of medical conditions, many often seen with aging, are discussed that may affect how safely and comfortably a person can exercise. Examples include: heart disease, pulmonary (lung) disease, osteoporosis, arthritis, fibromyalgia, diabetes, and obesity. Be sure to peruse the list of conditions to see if any apply to you.

Part Two: Doing It is where the action is. Page after page of both basic and specialized programs are assembled for warming up, muscle strengthening, balance, and stretching. Beginning or maintenance level, this manual is designed to be user-friendly and take the guesswork out of the endless exercise choices, providing something for everyone. Select programs that best fit your needs, and be sure to review the guidelines appropriate for you.

Appendix: Here to Help (Tools and References) is a collection of scales, logs/records, and references that make it easier and more meaningful for you to actually put your program into place. Find all the tools you need to be successful at aging fitfully. Feel free to make copies of logs and records.

HOW TO USE THE BOOK

Reading cover to cover: This is the best way to get a grasp of the big picture. However, chances are many of you will not read that way. For that reason, pertinent information often appears in more than one place. You will likely notice repetition of details. If you find yourself musing, "Haven't I read that somewhere before?"—chances are you have.

A little repetition, especially when it comes to exercise safety, never hurts. Additionally, many of the individual exercises appear in multiple places, as they have value under many circumstances and usefulness regarding many of the anticipated reader's goals.

Reading Specific Guidelines for Disabilities and Chronic Disease A to Z: Even if you would like to read the book cover to cover, the section covering specific conditions is probably not a section that an individual will read entirely. More likely, the medical conditions that have personal interest to the reader will receive the focus. The intent of this section is to provide enough information to be helpful, while not being overly scientific. This balance is difficult to achieve. If the information is too technical, find a resource or health professional that can help make it clearer. This section is printed on a different color paper, both for ease of accessibility and to set the depth and specific content apart from the rest of the book.

Using as a reference: This book has been organized to provide easy access to information. Readers may look up something specific about a medical condition or may go directly to exercise programs. It is highly recommended that enough time is spent reviewing guidelines to best ensure exercise safety.

TALKING ABOUT IT

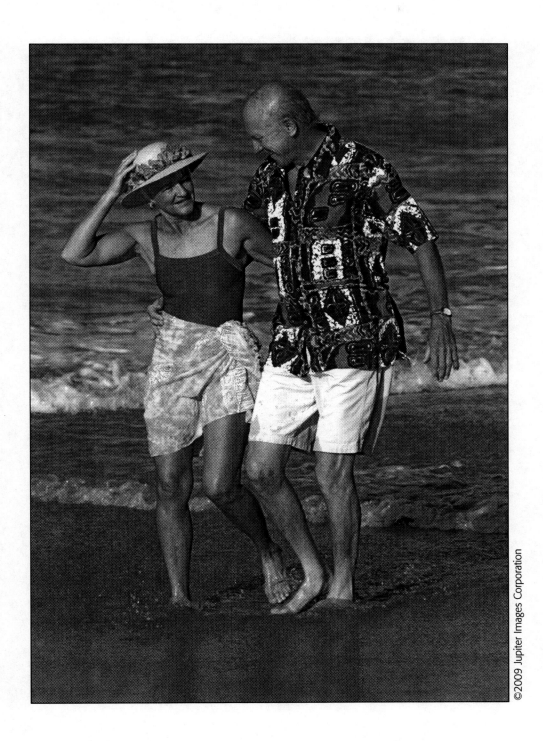

©2009 Jupiter Images Corporation

Part One

1

The Subtle Spiral Downward

Mom's Story...and Yours?

"Mom! You need to do something! You're *there*!"

I hung up the phone feeling anxious, surprised at what I'd just said, and worried about the implications of the discussion. Just what did I mean by *there*? I wasn't even sure myself. I had just spoken to my mother in North Dakota. She had been telling me about her excruciating knee pain, a chronic issue that had been getting increasingly worse. It was a classic case of adding insult to injury: a weakened, inflamed joint that routinely buckled under the stress of sudden movement. As is often the case, continual attempts to avoid pain in the knee had put more stress elsewhere. As a result, she was now aggravating a longtime heel spur on the other foot. Consequently, just getting around, much less going up and down stairs, was becoming almost impossible.

My mother, at 67 years old, was dealing with more than just pain. She was dealing with more than not being able to get around easily and take care of her home. She was faced with having to look for a less physically demanding job because, from a financial standpoint, she was unable to stop working. For a woman of almost 70 years with many physical limitations, viable employment options are dismal.

Mere Inconveniences...

An unfortunate story, yes, but admittedly a bit lukewarm in its level of drama. It lacks the power and emotions of far worse scenarios, disasters such as a sudden heart attack, a devastating stroke, or the dreaded discovery of cancer. A bad knee? Sure, that's sad, but...well, big deal, quite frankly.

Such is the insidious nature of seemingly mere inconveniences: the path they may lead us down does not look as bad as the path that some are forced to follow. Inconveniences are all too easy to dismiss—therein lies their power. They don't grab our attention like a heart attack. They don't make us suddenly grateful for survival or require us to fight for our lives. We can often tolerate and overlook them. And we do—sometimes for a very long time—until something else happens.

One month after that phone call, my mother fell. She simply stepped on an uneven surface in her bedroom. The good news was that she fell onto her bed. (What are the chances of that happening?) The bad news was that, in an instant, she completely ruptured her Achilles tendon to the degree that fragments of bone were torn from her heel. Her life had suddenly changed. Her job was no longer an issue—it was completely out of the question. Instead, she was faced with having surgery and going through a long rehabilitative period. She was even at risk of being sent to long-term care from the hospital instead of being able to go home. Long-term care was her worst fear.

Such is the insidious nature of seemingly mere inconveniences: they are all too easy to dismiss—therein lies their power.

Seemingly, one simple misstep changed everything—a stroke of bad luck. But is that really true? Likely, it had been several years of missteps that had made her increasingly vulnerable to such an ill-fated moment. During years, even decades, of being physically inactive, eating poorly, gaining weight, and not listening to the signs (or at least not taking them seriously), her body had accumulated the consequences of neglect.

The Average "Healthy" American

My mother's story is a fairly typical illustration of many people her age. She has been generally "healthy" most of her life (despite the fact that, like many Americans, she is considerably overweight, has high blood pressure, and suffers from arthritis). In our society, unfortunately, that scenario is pretty average. She would describe herself as having been fairly active in high school—she loved sports, but they weren't available for girls. She married and started having children right out of high school. It wouldn't be fair to call my mother sedentary during all those years of raising six children (I know we weren't easy), but she certainly didn't exercise per se. Like many women of her generation, she ran after kids, did lots *and lots* of laundry, cleaned house, and collapsed in front of the TV when the last child finally went to bed. As we grew up and left home, I think she welcomed the opportunity to *not* be running so much.

Fast forward a few decades. Ironically, that initial phone call about my mother's knee pain came as I was doing intense research for this book. I had been immersed for countless hours in the latest literature that continued to describe the effects of aging, the hazards of losing function, the downward spiral of deconditioning, and the risk of losing independence. All this literature was repeatedly countered with compelling research supporting the absolute necessity of combating these losses with exercise—not *just* into old age, but *especially* into old age.

Activities of daily living require sufficient strength no matter what your age: acts of pushing, pulling, lifting, climbing, carrying, reaching, stooping, bending, and walking. Research shows that most individuals who end up in nursing homes are not there because they are ill, but because they lack the fitness to maintain their independence. Other than not surviving, how can the stakes be higher?

"I Know I Should..."

When I emphatically told my mother "You *have* to do something," she heard what I was saying. She knew that she was *there*—at a place, physically, that she had been feeling herself approach but had been dealing with like the majority of people (i.e., seeking over-the-counter relief, prescribed anti-inflammatory medications, and even injections). These remedies had offered limited, temporary, or no relief. Her response to my suggestion of starting to exercise was a common one: *I know I should* (with a tone of guilt but without conviction). With this mindset, she spiraled further down the vicious cycle of disability and disuse. It is difficult to interrupt this cycle, especially when someone is finally experiencing its symptoms, because now it *hurts* to move.

Most individuals who end up in nursing homes are not there because they are ill, but because they lack the fitness to maintain their independence.

Part of the problem is that many of the losses that we experience with aging tend to accrue without our attention, and without affecting our daily lives. As many adults don't often call on themselves in physically challenging ways, it is easy for subtle changes in activity patterns to be largely masked before they become aware that anything has been lost. It may be that they cross a threshold into disability with a muscle or joint injury, like my mother, or with a diagnosis of a condition. Or, it may simply be that they try to participate in an activity that they are unaccustomed to doing (e.g., a hike or a bike ride) that leaves them unexpectedly short of breath or with surprising fatigue. Unfortunately, the response is often to avoid further physical activity, accompanied by that defeating adage: "What can I do? I'm just getting old."

My mother is now doing strengthening exercises every day, which she sheepishly admits are similar to the ones I've tried over the years to get her to do. She is feeling better, stronger, and more capable of getting around. She has a long road yet to go, but the loss of her independence staring her in the face was the wake-up call she needed. And, thankfully, she has answered the call.

Of course, it is preferable to wake up *before* disaster strikes, or unpleasant situations occur, or the constant, pervasive loss of energy prevents us from enjoying our lives—which is not to say that exercise will protect us from anything bad happening to our health. However, exercise may delay the onset of, reduce the symptoms of, and speed up the recovery from many health conditions to which we may be predisposed. In addition, it will just help us to feel better regardless of our life's circumstances.

The Slippery Slope

When you are about 30 years old, you cross an invisible but unavoidable line. That line is your biological peak. And while it varies from person to person, and indeed from function to function in our own bodies, our potential for fitness and physical function begins to decline. If you believe you are too young to be facing your decline, think again. Functionally, your body could be older—far older—than your biological age would warrant.

"What can I do? I'm just getting old."

The average loss of many bodily functions occurs at about two percent per year after the age of 30. With little physical activity, that translates to about 70 percent of loss of function by the time you are 90. How can you impact that outcome? Exercise, of course. Exercise can slow that loss to a half percent per year, resulting in that same 90-year-old body only losing 30 percent of its function. None of us can escape the potent effects of sedentary habits and aging. And too often—much too often—they go together. The converse is also true—everyone can benefit from a lifestyle of physical activity and exercise.

The question to ask ourselves as we approach (or are well into experiencing) the proverbial downhill slide is: How slippery will the slope be? Will it be something we coast down with the perception that age is happening to us? Or will we take full advantage of the opportunity we have to slow the decline, retain our abilities as long as we can, and enjoy the quality of the ride? Someone once said it best, "The goal is to die young at an old age."

Functional Fitness: "Do You Have What It Takes?"

To age fitfully, you must have a sufficient balance of "functional fitness." In other words, do you have what it takes to successfully meet your activities of daily living with minimal discomfort and a reserve of energy? It is alarming how many people teeter on the line of losing their occupations, their leisure activities, and, most seriously, their very independence because they lack functional fitness. Few people even recognize how close they really are to being in this situation. Consider the following statistics:

- For about half of those in their 70s, living independently is a maximum effort.
- Two-thirds of women over the age of 74 can't lift 10 pounds off the floor.
- The majority of individuals over the age of 75 can't walk fast enough across the street before the light changes.
- Thirty-five percent of all 65-year-olds and 50 percent of all 80-year-olds suffer from falls. Twenty to 60 percent are injured from those falls.
- Forty-five percent of women and 28 percent of men lack the shoulder flexibility necessary for daily living.

These statistics are powerful, but sometimes, the personal illustrations in daily living have the most impact. Successful functioning in real life can take on interesting definitions. Some examples of the kinds of comments I hear on a regular basis from people experiencing the benefits of fitness are as follows:

- "I was able to get to the second floor of my home for the first time in 10 years."
- "I put my coat on today and finally had no pain in my shoulder."
- "I can put my socks on without becoming short of breath."
- "I'm able to look over my shoulder while driving instead of pulling off the road."
- "I have enough energy to entertain my grandchildren all weekend."
- "I'm able to do my gardening without being exhausted the next day."
- "I can walk down the stairs normally, without having to stop on each step for fear of falling."

These triumphs may seem small, but they are really enormous successes that manifest themselves in dozens of ways. One of the first things you experience from becoming more fit is having more energy, a "symptom" that impacts everything. This side effect of exercise can highly enrich the quality of your life.

Exercise has side effects just like many medications. The most common is increased energy.

However, first and foremost, you've got to at least *meet* the daily demands. Climbing stairs, rising from a chair, getting out of a bathtub, opening windows, shopping for groceries, and crossing a street before the light changes are all activities that require sufficient fitness. Meeting your personal needs are the most basic activities of daily living. Taking care of your home and finances are fundamental activities of daily living. The fun stuff—the activities that really make life worth living—is what gets eliminated if you only have the energy to take care of your basic needs. Getting enough exercise will help ensure your ability to lead a rich, self-sufficient life, and it is your greatest medical insurance to preserve your physical function, freedom, and independence.

"I Get All the Exercise I Need." Physical Activity…or Exercise?

"I get all the exercise I need." That phrase is spoken frequently. Yet those words can describe remarkably different scenarios. On one hand, that comment is often followed by something like, "I am on the go all the time. I run a small farm (or take care of a big house, or do lots of gardening, or…you fill in the blank)." Often, these people do move around a great deal during their waking hours. They may rarely sit, but they may never go to a gym or go for an exercise walk. They are very *physically active*, but they don't *exercise*.

Compare that scenario to this common example, beginning with the same exact sentence: "I get all the exercise I need. I walk three times a week for 30 minutes at a time with my heart rate in its target training zone." To their credit, the people who make this kind of statement are successfully following a fairly standard exercise recommendation. However, when you look at the rest of their waking hours, they may be quite sedentary. Perhaps they have inactive hobbies or a desk job. At any rate, they do exercise regularly, but other than the 90 total minutes of walking per week, they don't move around much. They *exercise*, but are not very *physically active*.

These two examples are illustrations of physical activity versus exercise. The two terms are often interchangeable, but they do have an important distinction. Defined simply:

Are you physically active but don't exercise? Or do you exercise but aren't physically active? Which is better?

> Physical activity = movement—any and all movement
> Exercise = structured movement

Exercise is a form of physical activity. It is planned and has intention. Usually, the intention is to become more fit. Therefore, physical activity is the "umbrella" term: it may or may not be exercise. So, who is better off: the person who is physically active but doesn't exercise? Or the person who exercises but is not physically active?

First, they are both better off than most. Doing *something* is almost always better than doing *nothing*. However, what appears to be true is that a combination of both physical activity and exercise is most beneficial. Just being more physically active has positive health impacts, while exercise best ensures a balance of fitness, as described in the next section.

Striking a Balance: The Fitness Tripod

Fitness is primarily comprised of three components, and can be thought of as a tripod. If all three legs are not well in place, the tripod is wobbly and at risk of falling. The three legs of fitness are identified and described in Figure 1-1. A more detailed version appears in Appendix A.

Tripod Leg #1: Aerobic Exercise for the Heart

Aerobic exercise is probably the most commonly known form of exercise. For many who consider themselves "successful exercisers," such as regular walkers, aerobic exercise is often what they are actually doing. Aerobic exercise is known to improve *cardiovascular endurance*, or the body's ability to take in, transport, and utilize oxygen efficiently. A standard "prescription" for aerobic exercise (based on the American College of Sports Medicine recommendations) is shown in Table 1-1.

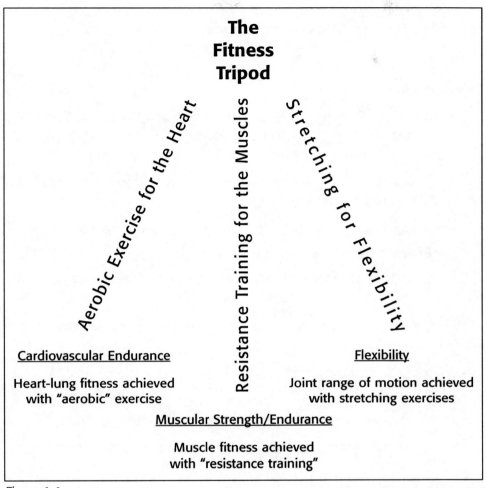

Figure 1-1

Ideally, a well-balanced exercise program should address all three components of fitness: aerobic exercise for cardiovascular fitness, resistance training for muscular strength and muscular endurance, and stretching for better flexibility.

Individuals who are at low fitness levels, very sedentary, older, diseased, or disabled should do the following:

- Read the "Exercise Safety" section later in this chapter.
- Consider seeing your physician before beginning. Complete the PAR-Q (Physical Activity Readiness Questionnaire) in Appendix B for recommendations.
- Perform lower-intensity exercise, i.e., fairly light (11) to somewhat hard (13) on the Rating of Perceived Exertion (RPE) scale (see Table 1-2). In some cases, especially when just starting or if you are very unfit, it is appropriate and effective to do exercise that is very light (9-10) on the RPE scale.

Aerobic Exercise: Standard Prescription

Frequency: 3-5 days per week

Intensity: Moderate to vigorous

- Moderate = Fairly light (11) to somewhat hard (13) on the Rating of Perceived Exertion (RPE) scale (Table 1-2)
  - ✓Example: Walking a 15- to 20-minute mile
    - ✓50-70% of estimated maximum heart rate (see "Heart Rate" in this chapter and page 143)
- Vigorous = Somewhat hard (13) to hard (15) on the RPE scale
  - ✓Example: Walking a 12-minute mile
    - ✓70-85% of estimated maximum heart rate (see "Heart Rate" in this chapter and page 143)

Duration: 20-60 minutes, continuous or intermittent (increasing to 10- to 15-minute bouts)

Mode of Exercise: Rhythmical movement of large muscle groups

Examples: Walking, jogging, bicycling (stationary or outdoor), rowing, swimming*/water exercise, hiking, dancing, and cross-county skiing

*Horizontal swimming will result in lower aerobic heart rates, on average 10-12 beats per minute lower than upright exercise.

Table 1-1. Aerobic exercise: standard prescription

- Perform multiple sessions of short duration (1 to 10 minutes, depending on capability), gradually increasing the time of each session and decreasing the frequency of sessions per day as fitness improves. For example, you may start by doing four five-minute sessions throughout the day, and progress to doing two 10-minute bouts, increasing to two 15-minute sessions, and finally one 30-minute session.

Individuals who are at higher fitness levels should do the following:

- Read the "Exercise Safety" section later in this chapter.
- Perform higher intensity exercise to improve or maintain fitness (somewhat hard (13) to hard (15) on the RPE scale).
- Caution: High intensity aerobic exercise, while resulting in the greatest health and fitness returns, is sometimes associated with lower adherence and a higher risk of heart and orthopedic injuries, particularly if vigorous exercise is not done regularly. Be sure to increase in a gradually progressive manner, be consistent, and pay attention to symptoms. If you develop cardiac or

joint/muscle symptoms, reduce or discontinue your exercise and consult a professional. (For a list of symptoms, see "What is your level of risk?").

Monitoring Your Aerobic Exercise Intensity

You can use several methods to help ensure that you are exercising within a safe, effective range:

- *Heart rate:* Heart rate is often used to monitor aerobic exercise intensity. The most accurate method is by using results from a maximum stress test administered by a professional. Since the majority of people don't have that information available to them, a "target exercise heart rate" can be estimated by simple calculations. These estimations can have a relatively large margin of error, so it is important to also monitor your effort level (see Table 1-2) and your symptoms. Also be aware that some medications can affect heart rate. Ask your physician if you are taking anything that can increase or decrease your heart rate. Consult the "Monitoring Exercise Intensity With Heart Rate" section in Appendix C for commonly recommended exercise heart rate guidelines, as well as how to locate and count your pulse.

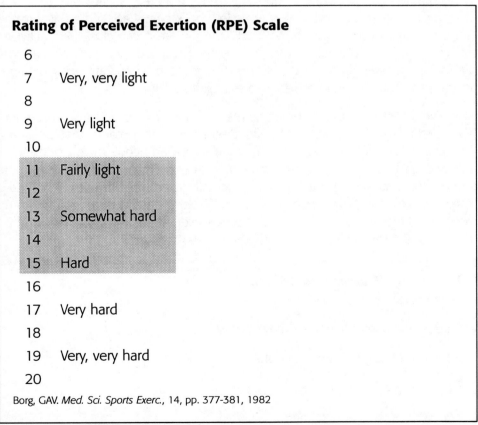

Rating of Perceived Exertion (RPE) Scale

6	
7	Very, very light
8	
9	Very light
10	
11	Fairly light
12	
13	Somewhat hard
14	
15	Hard
16	
17	Very hard
18	
19	Very, very hard
20	

Borg, GAV. *Med. Sci. Sports Exerc.*, 14, pp. 377-381, 1982

Table 1-2. Rating of perceived exertion (RPE) scale

• *Rating of Perceived Exertion (RPE) Scale* (Table 1-2): This subjective scale (Borg, GAV. *Med. Sci. Sports Exerc.*, 14, pp. 377-381, 1982) is a valuable and reliable way to monitor your intensity. It is referred to frequently in this book. It allows you to rate your overall effort level during exercise. The scale ranges from 6 to 20, or from rest (very, very light) to maximum effort (very, very hard). The usual recommendations for safe, effective exercise intensity range from 11 to 15, or at least fairly light but not more than hard. The RPE scale also appears in Appendix D.

In summary, the general recommendation (based on the surgeon general's report, *Physical Activity and Health*, 1996) is to accumulate at least 30 minutes of moderate-level physical activity (11 to 13 on the RPE scale) on most days of the week. Strive for more vigorous physical activity (14 to 15 on the RPE scale) if your health condition is stable and you tolerate your exercise with no symptoms. Be sure to complete the PAR-Q in Appendix B for guidance on your readiness to exercise.

Tripod Leg #2: Stretching for Flexibility

Stretching exercises help to optimize flexibility, or range of motion, in all the joints. Flexibility is particularly important in the hip area, as lack of flexibility in that location is associated with chronic low back pain. Lack of flexibility in the shoulders, upper and lower torso, neck, and hip areas can also affect activities of daily living. Risk of falling can be greatly increased with lack of sufficient flexibility. Interestingly, a loss of muscle strength, combined with aging changes in the joint, can also lead to reduced overall flexibility.

The safest and easiest stretching method to learn is called *static stretching* (i.e., getting into a position of mild discomfort and holding that position). Stretching exercises can be included in warm-ups and cool-downs, or done as a stand-alone activity. However, light, rhythmic physical activities should be done before stretching exercises to sufficiently warm the muscles. A standard "prescription" for flexibility is shown in Table 1-3. Examples of warm-up programs appear in Chapter 3. For more detailed stretching guidelines and an outline of the various stretching programs, see Chapter 5.

Flexibility: Standard Prescription
(see exercises in Chapter 5)

Frequency: Minimum of 2-3 days per week

Intensity: Mild discomfort (should not be painful)

Duration: 10-30 seconds

Repetitions: 1-4 for each stretch

Mode of Exercise: Stretching for all major muscle groups and joints

---

Table 1-3. Flexibility: standard prescription

Tripod Leg #3: Resistance Training for the Muscles

The primary focus of this book is on resistance training. Resistance training involves methodically and progressively exerting muscles against a load. It is commonly known as weight lifting or weight training. Resistance training improves and maintains muscular fitness. Since all movement requires muscles, a sufficient level of muscular strength (the ability to lift a given load) and muscular endurance (the ability to do work over time) is critical. Muscle power (the ability to quickly contract the muscle forcefully) is probably most related to activities of daily living such as getting out of a chair, climbing steps, etc.

Resistance training provides health benefits that are extensive and profound. Furthermore, the need for resistance training not only continues as you get older, it becomes even more important. An average of 30 percent of muscle strength is lost between the ages of 50 and 70, and losses beyond age 80 are even greater.

Does everyone need resistance training? Yes. Well, almost everyone. In a few instances, resistance training would not be beneficial (see "Resistance Training With Disabilities and Chronic Diseases" in Chapter 2). But, the vast majority of people stand to greatly benefit from resistance training.

Resistance Training: Standard Prescription
(see exercises in Chapter 4)

Frequency: 2-3 days per week on nonconsecutive days (i.e., spread it out)

Intensity: Moderate to vigorous

- Moderate = Somewhat hard (12-13) on the RPE Scale
- Vigorous = Hard to very hard (15-17) on the RPE Scale, only if tolerated safely (see Table 1-2)

Repetitions: 1-3 sets of 8-15 (see more specific guidelines in Chapter 1)

Examples: Elastic bands or tubing, hand weights/barbells, resistance machines

Note: Be sure to read Chapter 2 for help in modifying these recommendations based on your individual needs.

Table 1-4. Resistance training: standard prescription

A Balancing Act:
Balance and the Fitness Tripod

Balance is the ability to maintain your body's center of gravity over the base of support. It is an important part of functional fitness. Impaired balance increases the risk of falling. Between the ages of 60 and 85, the risk of falling for women is 75 percent. Falls are responsible for 95 percent of hip fractures. So, why is balance not a part of the tripod (aside from the obvious fact that a tripod has only three legs and wouldn't be a tripod with a fourth leg)?

The protective effect of exercise appears to increase with age.

The answer is because balance abilities are largely associated with the three fitness components that have been discussed in this chapter. The better your aerobic fitness, muscular strength/endurance, and flexibility, the better your balance. Increased fitness improves walking speed, walking distance, and stride length. In fact, women reporting more than one mile per day of walking have a 50 percent lower risk of falling.

Multiple additional factors are associated with balance problems, including vision disorders, inner ear disorders, attention challenges, and medical conditions. The medical conditions often associated with balance issues include stroke, arthritis, cardiovascular disease, osteoporosis, Parkinson's disease, and diabetes. Exercise can reduce balance risks imposed by these conditions by improving disease status, increasing confidence and attention abilities, and reducing medication needs.

The types and number of medications being taken can also affect balance. Studies show that older adults taking more than four prescription medications are more at risk for falling. Antidepressant medications in particular increase the risk of falling, especially for new users and those on higher dosages. Given the well-known fact that exercise can improve mood, the risk of falling can potentially be reduced by decreasing or eliminating the need for antidepressants.

Balance: Standard Prescription
(see exercises in Chapter 6)

Frequency: 2-3 days per week

Duration: 10-30 seconds per position (start with 5-15 seconds)

Repetitions: 1 set of each balance exercise

Mode of Exercise: 5-10 exercises, starting with the "Beginning Program" (see Chapter 6)

Table 1-5. Balance: standard prescription

What's In It for Me?
Benefits of Exercise/Regular Physical Activity

You (and your body) will enjoy many benefits from an exercise and regular physical activity program. The benefits include:

- Improved heart and lung function

- Reduced coronary artery disease risk factors such as lower blood pressure, healthier blood cholesterol profile, lower body fat, reduced need for insulin, and better blood sugar control. (Because older adults have been alive for a longer period of time, they have a longer exposure to these risk factors. Unfortunately, aging also results in a reduced ability to cope with these factors, which is a compelling reason for older adults to exercise.)

- Lower mortality (death) and morbidity (illness) from diseases such as cardiovascular diseases, some cancers, and Type II diabetes (This benefit is both from a prevention level, i.e., primary prevention, and also from a rehabilitative level when these disease conditions are already present, i.e., secondary prevention.)

- Less anxiety and depression, an enhanced sense of well-being, and improved work, recreational, and sport performance

Current evidence (according to ACSM) indicates that exercise may also be beneficial in *decreasing* the risk of other chronic diseases:

- The evidence is *excellent* relating exercise to: all-cause mortality, coronary artery disease, and colon cancer.

- The evidence is *good* relating exercise to: hypertension, obesity, Type II diabetes, and osteoporosis.

- *Some* evidence exists relating exercise to: stroke and cancers of the breast, prostate, and lung.

- There appears to be no apparent difference relating exercise to: peripheral vascular disease (blood flow problems in legs), cancers of the rectum, stomach, and pancreas, and osteoarthritis.

Taking a Risk?
Exercise Safety

If heart disease is not already present, the risk involved in exercising is extremely low. In general, risk of cardiovascular complications is lowest for young, healthy adults and nonsmoking women. The risk increases for people with multiple risk factors and people experiencing symptoms (see "What is your level of risk?"). Risk is highest in those with established heart disease. As stated in *ACSM's Guidelines for Exercise Testing and Prescription 6th ed.*

(2000), "regardless of the presence or absence of heart disease, the overall absolute risk of cardiovascular complications during exercise is low, especially when weighed against the associated health benefits." In fact, findings suggest regular exercise provides protection against heart attack and cardiac arrest, even during vigorous exercise, as well as other times.

What Is Your Level of Risk?

- Review the following lists to help identify your risk level, and see where you fall in: "Initial ACSM Risk Stratification" levels shown in Table 1-6.
  - ✓ Risk Factors for Coronary Artery Disease
    - ⇨ Family history
    - ⇨ Diabetes
    - ⇨ Cigarette smoking
    - ⇨ Obesity
    - ⇨ High blood pressure (hypertension)
    - ⇨ Sedentary lifestyle
    - ⇨ High blood cholesterol
    - ⇨ Age
  - ✓ Potential Major Signs and Symptoms of Cardiovascular/Pulmonary Disease
    - ⇨ Pain in chest, neck, jaw, arms
    - ⇨ Shortness of breath at rest or during mild exertion
    - ⇨ Dizziness/fainting
    - ⇨ Ankle swelling
    - ⇨ "Funny" heartbeats (palpitations)
    - ⇨ "Racing" heart rate
    - ⇨ Unexplained anxiety, weakness, fatigue
    - ⇨ Unusual fatigue or shortness of breath with usual activities
    - ⇨ Known heart murmur
    - ⇨ Nausea or vomiting
    - ⇨ Unusual sweating with usual activities
    - ⇨ Pain in calves/thighs with exercise (especially walking) that ceases when exercise is stopped
- Be sure to complete the PAR-Q (Physical Activity Readiness Questionnaire) in Appendix B. The questionnaire will help you decide whether or not you should see your physician before you begin an exercise program.
- Risk of *cardiovascular (heart)* complications associated with exercise further *increases* if:

Initial ACSM Risk Stratification

Low risk: Young (men age 44 or younger; women age 54 or younger), no symptoms, no more than one risk factor (see "What is your level of risk?")

Moderate risk: Older (men age 45 or older; women age 55 or older), two or more risk factors (see "What is your level of risk?")

High risk: One or more signs/symptoms (see "What is your level of risk?") or known cardiovascular, pulmonary, or metabolic disease (diabetes, thyroid, renal, or liver disease)

Table 1-6. Initial ACSM risk stratification

✓ Exercise is relatively infrequent (less than three times per week) and inconsistent (risk is especially increased with less than one session per week).

✓ Exercise intensity is unfamiliar and inappropriate (more than mild/moderate for older, deconditioned, and/or people with chronic disease; more than vigorous for young and/or healthy individuals). When progressing, *do not do much more than you are accustomed to* (increases of no more than 5 to 15 percent per week or every other week). See previous guidelines in Tripod Leg #1.

✓ Routine warming up and cooling down are not included in exercise session (risk goes up when exercise is suddenly and abruptly initiated and/or suddenly ceased).

• Risk of *musculoskeletal (muscle/joint)* injury *increases* with:

✓ Excessive frequency of exercise (greater than five days a week)

✓ Long durations (greater than 45 minutes)

✓ High intensities (greater than an RPE of 13 or somewhat hard) (see Table 1-2)

✓ Improper exercise technique

✓ Pre-existing joint instability or history of injury

✓ Lack of variety in exercise program

✓ Avoidance of appropriate warm-ups and cool-downs

(Also see Chapter 2, beginning with "What if I become injured or have previous joint/muscle pain?").

Note: To help you monitor your weekly physical activity and make sure you are getting variety, a balance of structured exercise, and wise pacing, make copies of the Physical Activity Record in Appendix O (a completed sample for reference appears in Appendix P). Documenting can help reveal patterns you may not otherwise observe, as well as keep you more accountable. Even if you are not inclined to do paperwork, *try it.*

2

Resistance Training

In the Spotlight: Resistance Training Takes Center Stage

As previously mentioned, resistance training receives special focus in this book. The primary reason is because of its potential health value (see the following list of benefits). In fact, the importance of resistance training has been so widely recognized that the surgeon general, as well as most major health organizations, recommends resistance training as part of a total exercise program. Organizations sharing this recommendation include the American College of Sports Medicine (ACSM), the American Heart Association (AHA), and the American Association for Cardiovascular and Pulmonary Rehabilitation (AACVPR).

The second major reason resistance training is taking the spotlight in this book is because most people do not recognize its benefits or do not incorporate it into a regular routine. The percentage of the general population actually *doing* resistance training speaks to a need for greater awareness: *only 20 percent of men and less than 9 percent of women report participating in any kind of muscle strengthening exercise.* These numbers are even lower in the older adult population who would benefit the most. Despite the high safety and effectiveness record, even for the frail elderly, only 6 percent of people between the ages of 65 and 74, 4 percent of people over the age of 75, and an estimated fewer than 1 percent of people over the age of 85 are actually doing resistance training. Furthermore, fewer women than men participate in resistance training at all ages...even though they begin losing strength at an earlier age and a faster rate than men.

Only 20 percent of men and less than 9 percent of women report participating in any kind of muscle strengthening exercise. This percentage is far less in older adults (1 to 6 percent), even though they need it the most.

The important benefits of resistance training include the following:

- Increased muscle strength, muscle mass, and muscle endurance
- Improved neuromuscular (nerve-muscle) coordination

- Modest improvements in cardiovascular endurance (3 to 12 percent)
- Improved bone mineral density (reducing the risk or severity of osteoporosis)
- Favorable shift in body composition (lower body fat and higher fat-free mass)
- Lowered blood pressure (in people with high blood pressure)
- Improved insulin/blood sugar control (important for diabetics)
- Improved blood lipids (blood fat/cholesterol) profile
- Reduced risk of orthopedic (muscle/joint) injuries and treatment for injuries
- Less low back pain
- Improved functional capacity (the ability to perform the activities of daily living)
- Less load on the heart during daily activities
- Lowered risk of falling in older adults
- Increased walking distance and speed with improved gait
- Improved sense of well-being
- Better quality of life

Isn't Walking All I Need?

A common misconception is to think that a single kind of exercise can sufficiently provide you with all the most important components of fitness. Walking is good for you—if you are currently walking as a regular form of exercise, don't give it up. But walking is primarily an aerobic exercise, and, thus, doesn't provide everything you need to be considered fit.

Walking doesn't appreciably improve muscle strength, muscle mass, or bone mineral density (see the section on osteoporosis later in this chapter), which are all critical aspects of fitness. You need *resistance training* to improve muscle fitness. Balance training and flexibility training, while important in your overall program, does little to improve muscle mass or strength.

Resistance training is the most effective way to counter the losses of muscle mass associated with aging, estimated to be 20 to 50 percent over the adult life span.

Resistance training is the most effective way to counter the losses of muscle mass associated with aging, which is estimated to be 20 to 50 percent over the adult life span (30 percent between the ages of 50 and 70). Moreover, resistance training improves *all* of the essential fitness components of physical function: muscle strength, muscle endurance, balance, and flexibility. Supplementing your walking (or other aerobic exercise) program with resistance training and stretching will provide a sufficient balance of fitness.

Can't Resistance Training Be Kind of Dangerous?

Resistance training, when performed according to guidelines and with proper form, is actually quite safe. With regard to heart-related incidents, resistance training has a remarkable safety record. Extensive research on many thousands of participants has failed to find a single report on fatal incidents. Even in patients with known coronary artery disease, including stage II and stage III congestive heart failure, no events have been reported.

This statistic may be attributable in part to the fact that resistance training is typically done in sets that are completed in one to two minutes and interspersed with rests. This style is in contrast with aerobic exercise, which can last 20 continuous minutes or more.

Musculoskeletal injuries, such as ligament sprains, muscle strains, or fractures, can occur with resistance training. These kinds of injuries happen more frequently with high-level training and when improper body mechanics or techniques are used. However, the single greatest risk of experiencing these kinds of injuries is when a history of a previous injury exists.

The single greatest cause of musculoskeletal (muscle/joint) injury with resistance training is when a history of a previous injury exists.

But What if I Have a Disease, Chronic Condition, or I'm Just too Old?

First of all, regarding the age factor...*nonsense*. You are never too old. Studies have shown dramatic improvements in strength in frail people in their 90s. In fact, older adults seem to reap the most dramatic improvements with resistance training—studies have shown ranges of 25 to 174 percent (25 to 30 percent is similar to the normal loss of muscle strength in 30 years of aging). With the functional decline, heightened risk of falling, and the potential loss of independence in older adults, no time in your life is more critical to be exercising, *including doing resistance training*. Even if you have *never* exercised before, you can start benefiting from resistance training now.

Women should pay particular attention to resistance training. Studies have shown half of all women over the age of 65 can't lift 10 pounds. In fact, women start losing strength at an earlier age and a faster rate compared to men. Despite women's longer life span, on average, compared to men, studies have shown women are more susceptible to becoming frail and spending more of their later years in dependent living (eight years, on average, versus three years for men).

Older adults see the most dramatic improvements with resistance training—a whopping range of 25 to 174 percent.

Secondly, if you have a chronic disease or a medical condition, chances are that resistance training, along with a well-balanced exercise program, will come highly recommended based on the latest research. While an exercise program may not cure a disease or make a condition go away, it often helps people cope with that disease or condition more constructively. Exercise can improve quality of life, as well as help people retain the ability to live independently. Estimates show that when aging is coupled with a chronic disease, the risk of dependent living triples. So...is it safe to resistance train? Perhaps a better question is: Is it safe not to?

What if I Become Injured or Have Previous Joint/Muscle Pain?

Having an injury or disability can be a barrier to becoming more physically active, especially if you are older or overweight. If you already have pain and have had it longer than two weeks, consult your physician to have it evaluated. Avoid exercises or ranges of motion that aggravate the pain. (If you have arthritis, fibromyalgia, or other degenerative joint disease, see the section Resistance Training With Disabilities and Chronic Diseases later in this chapter.)

Half of all women over the age of 65 can't lift 10 pounds.

Injury is more likely to occur with *unaccustomed* exercise (i.e., exercise that is more or different than what you have been doing physically in the past three months on a *regular* basis), especially when strain exceeds your current limits. The following tips will further reduce your risk of becoming injured or aggravating an old injury.

Tips to Reduce the Risk of Injury With Resistance Training

- Use caution when you begin, starting with little, or no, added resistance.
- Enlist guidance from a trained professional who can design your program based on your needs and supervise your sessions (at least in the beginning to get you started).
- Pay attention to your technique—proper form is a must. Practice exercises in front of a mirror.
- Move through the range of motion of your exercises slowly and with control, stopping before you feel pain.

Is it safe to resistance train? Perhaps a better question is: *Is it safe not to?*

- Perform a light, active warm-up before exercising (e.g., walking in place), which will increase the tissue temperature (along with other favorable metabolic changes). Performing stretches after light physical activity is fine during a warm-up, but no evidence suggests it will help to prevent injury. Stretches during a cool-down are more effective and will help improve your overall range of motion.
- Vary your routine. Exercising in the same way day after day, especially without enough recovery time, increases the risk of injury. Cross-training is a great idea. Intersperse a variety of aerobic activities around your resistance training program, or vary how you do the same aerobic exercise from day to day (i.e., take shorter, faster walks on the days you resistance train, and take longer, slower walks on the days in between). This variation also helps you avoid getting bored.
- Avoid doing too much too soon, a common risk when you start feeling better. Allow at least 48 hours of recovery time between resistance training sessions.
- As a general guideline, do not increase resistance training exercise (frequency, intensity, or duration) by more than 2 to 10 percent each week (for more details, see How Fast (or Slowly) Should I Progress With Resistance Training? later in this chapter).

- Practice the *hard/easy principle* with your overall exercise program. Doing so means always interspersing harder days with easier days, not necessarily taking every other day off from exercise altogether. It may mean alternating activities and reducing the duration or intensity of exercise. For some, especially older or more deconditioned people, doing resistance training and aerobic activities on separate days works well.

If You Develop Pain or Injury With Resistance Training

- Rest the injured area for a couple of days.

- Apply ice to the injured area frequently (a minimum of two to three times a day for a period of 20 to 30 minutes). Apply ice with compression and elevate when possible. If using gel packs, rotate between at least two, keeping one in the freezer to keep the cold temperature more consistent.

- Avoid trying to work through the pain, which will only aggravate the injury and make it harder to resolve in the long run. In addition, an injury may alter the way you do your normal activities, putting unaccustomed stress on other joints/tissue, possibly resulting in a second injury.

- Avoid any exercises that aggravate the pain. Seek guidance to modify painful exercises or find appropriate substitutes.

- Get a medical evaluation of any pain that persists longer than two weeks. To better describe and identify pain or discomfort to your doctor or another health professional, consult the Rating of Pain Scale in Appendix D.

GETTING SPECIFIC: RESISTANCE TRAINING GUIDELINES

Basic resistance training guidelines were discussed in Chapter 1. The following section provides more specific information regarding what is necessary for a safe, effective resistance training program. The information comes primarily from the American College of Sports Medicine (ACSM), the leading authority on exercise-related guidelines.

Most people who are beginning an exercise program want to know one thing, *How much do I have to do?* In other words, what is the minimal amount needed for sufficient improvement? The majority of us don't want to have to invest a great deal of time, no matter how convinced we are that it's good for us. In fact, part of the reason why so few people have participated in resistance training may be because of the misconception that it will take a lot of time.

Studies show that programs that exceed an hour in duration are associated with a high drop-out rate. Fortunately, a solid, well-rounded resistance training program shouldn't take longer than 15 to 30 minutes. Avoid time-consuming, labor-intensive, and complicated programs. They aren't necessary.

Basic Resistance Training Guidelines

Guidelines for Healthy Adults Under 50 to 60 Years of Age

Generally speaking, muscular *strength* is enhanced when a higher resistance (load) is coupled with few repetitions (six or less). Lower resistance (load) with high repetitions (20 or more) has the greatest effect on muscular *endurance*. Put another way:

High load + low reps = greater muscle strength
Low load + high reps = greater muscle endurance

A program designed to fall somewhere in the middle provides a combination of both. Current resistance training recommendations for healthy adults (Table 2-1) strive to improve both muscular strength and endurance.

Guidelines for Healthy Adults Under 50 to 60 Years of Age

How many? Eight to ten exercises using all major muscle groups (arms, chest, abdomen, back, hips, and legs).

How much? One to three sets of 8 to 12 repetitions of each exercise.

How often? Two to three times per week (48 hours recovery is appropriate).

How hard? Initial intensity goal should be comfortably hard (RPE 12 to 13, somewhat hard), progressing gradually to higher intensity (RPE 15 to 17, hard to very hard).

Note: The greatest benefits over the long term occur when effort is gradually increased to an RPE of 19 to 20, maximal, *if safely tolerated.* (RPE of 19 to 20 is achieved when, upon completing your last repetition, you could not complete another repetition in good form.) Gradually increase the repetitions or resistance at this level every one to two weeks until you reach a maintenance level. Add variation for best results.

Table 2-1. Guidelines for healthy adults under 50 to 60 years of age

Guidelines for Healthy Adults 50 to 60+ Years of Age or More Frail Individuals

The general principles for resistance training apply to older adults or more frail individuals. However, compared to younger, healthy people, older adults and more frail individuals should perform more repetitions at a lighter resistance. This method reduces the risk of injury and may improve tolerance. This method is also appropriate for people at any age who are more interested in focusing on muscle endurance versus muscle strength. Also, progression should be slower in older adults. Refer to Table 2-2 for the complete resistance training guidelines for healthy adults 50 to 60+ years of age or more frail individuals.

Guidelines for Healthy Adults 50 to 60+ Years of Age or More Frail Individuals

How many? Eight to ten exercises using all major muscle groups (arms, chest, abdomen, back, hips, and legs). Consider choosing just two to three upper body and two to three lower body exercises to start.

How much? One set minimum of 10 to 15 repetitions of each exercise—may increase very gradually to two or three sets as tolerated and if desired.

How often? Two to three times per week. (A longer recovery period is even more important in older adults—only twice a week may be more appropriate in some circumstances.)

How hard? Intensity can be moderate initially (RPE 12 to 13, somewhat hard). Progress more slowly than younger adults, gradually adding repetitions or resistance every two to four weeks to allow time for adaptation. With toleration, older adults can safely increase intensity to a feeling of muscle fatigue. If returning from a layoff, start with an intensity of approximately half your previously-used resistance, and gradually build back up to pre-layoff levels.

Table 2-2. Guidelines for healthy adults 50 to 60+ years of age or more frail individuals

How Fast Will I Get Strong?

Increases in strength happen surprisingly fast. The greatest strength gains will take place in the first four to eight weeks, and will occur to the greatest degree in untrained or deconditioned individuals. Increases are less dramatic for more fit people. Studies ranging from four weeks to two years show an average of 40 percent strength increase in people who have not exercised, compared to only 2 percent for elite athletes. Improvements in strength observed in the first month are attributed primarily to changes in the nervous system that lead to greater coordination with the exercises. Beyond the first month, strength gains are due primarily to an increase in muscle size, a phenomenon called *hypertrophy*.

These strength increases seem to be similar in the beginning whether resistance training is performed in single-set or multiple-set (two to three) programs. The degree of improvement between one set compared to multiple sets in the first three to four months is minimal (about 3 to 5 percent). Similarly, studies show that 80 to 90 percent of the resistance training benefits can be obtained in two days per week versus three days per week of training for beginners. Therefore, for most of the adult population, one set of resistance training exercises performed two days a week is sufficient for the first three months.

Similarly, it doesn't seem to take much resistance to improve maximum strength in sedentary individuals. Even loads of 45 to 50 percent of one's maximum strength levels (roughly equivalent to about an RPE of 9 to 11, very light to fairly light), and in some cases even less, are sufficient to improve strength initially.

How Do I Progress With Resistance Training?

The following information comes primarily from ACSM's position statement on progression guidelines for healthy adults (2002). Read on for more information relating to chronic disease and disability.

Strength gains slow as resistance training is continued. Progression is needed to continue to improve muscular strength. This principle is called the *overload principle* and applies to all individuals, fit or unfit, young or old. Progress can mean increasing overall volume or adding variety. This criteria can be met by:

- Adding more repetitions
- Adding more resistance
- Doing multiple sets
- Utilizing rest periods
- Changing the order, or sequence, of exercises performed
- Changing the selection of exercises performed
- Using other variation approaches (e.g., periodization)

Adding More Repetitions

In general, it is recommended that repetitions be added before resistance, especially for older adults. If you are a healthy individual, younger than 50 to 60 years of age, and on an 8-to-12 repetitions program, increase repetitions to 12 before adding resistance and reducing to eight repetitions. If you are on a 10-to-15 repetitions program, which is recommended for older adults, increase repetitions to 15 before adding resistance and reducing to 10 repetitions.

Adding More Resistance

Adding more resistance is recommended as resistance training continues, increasing to 60 to 80 percent of maximum strength (roughly equivalent to about an RPE of 12 to 13, somewhat hard to 15, hard). Long-term resistance training for advanced, younger, healthy individuals using 80 to 100 percent (RPE 19 to 20) and incorporating variety will maximize strength improvements.

(Be aware that the risk of injury and the risk of not being compliant over the long term increases with this level of training.)

Doing Multiple Sets

Performing one set of an exercise is a minimum guideline. Going beyond one set will further improve strength levels after the initial three months of consistent resistance training. Increase to two sets, and if well tolerated, you may choose to increase to three. *It is important to note that you do not have to perform the same number of sets for each exercise.* You may choose to do two to three sets for areas of concern or interest, and one to two sets for just basic fitness.

Utilizing Rest Periods

When doing multiple sets, rest periods between sets are important. The amount of rest can significantly affect the way your body responds to your exercise. If rest periods are too short, strength increases can be compromised. This concept demonstrates the importance of recovery with strength training.

Shorter rest periods are usually associated with more *muscular endurance* improvement (between sets of exercises performed with higher repetitions and lower loads). Longer rest periods (between sets of exercises performed with lower repetitions and higher loads) are usually associated with greater *muscular strength* increases.

In general, rest periods of two to three minutes are appropriate for exercises that use heavier loads, larger muscle groups, and multiple joints. Rest periods of one to two minutes are appropriate for those exercises using lesser loads, smaller muscle groups, and single joints. For older adults, one- to two-minute rest periods are usually sufficient.

Changing the Order, or Sequence, of Exercises Performed

Simply changing the order of exercises can favorably impact how your body responds to the exercises. Be mindful of general sequencing guidelines (e.g., working larger muscle groups before smaller ones, doing multiple-joint exercises before single-joint exercises, and rotating upper and lower body). With those guidelines in mind, be sure to mix up your routine.

Changing the Selection of Exercises Performed

Your body will respond to variation in the exercises selected. (See the Maintenance #1 and Maintenance #2 programs in Chapter 4.) Rotating back and forth between programs every two to three months will encourage more improvement than doing the same exercises in the same way over a long period of time.

Using Other Variation Approaches (e.g., Periodization)

The subject of periodization is usually reserved for serious weight lifters. However, this well-established way to vary resistance training programs over the long term clearly supports the principle of variety. Some younger, healthy adults may want to incorporate at least some form of "periodizing" after a good foundation is established with an initial three to six months of consistent resistance training following the basic guidelines, and older adults may still benefit from including modified variations of this principle.

In general, periodizing systematically varies training volume and intensity from session to session. While most often associated with elite athletes, periodization has been used successfully with individuals of many fitness levels involved in recreational exercise, and even for those rehabilitating from injury.

Many forms of periodization can be used. One that may interest the readers of this book, especially if you are healthy, under 60 years of age, and have established a solid, consistent resistance training base, is a modified approach that is incorporated over the week. For a three-day-a-week program (e.g., Monday, Wednesday, and Friday), randomly use heavier resistance with fewer repetitions (five to six) on one day, moderate resistance and moderate repetitions (8 to 10) on the next training day, and lighter resistance with higher repetitions (12 to 15) on the third day.

While this approach isn't necessarily a *recommendation* for older adults, some variation could be safely and effectively incorporated, perhaps by doing fewer repetitions (8 to 10) with a little more resistance on some days, and doing a few more repetitions (12 to 15) at a lighter resistance on other days. The point is that variation is important to include in your program over the long term—after a solid, consistent foundation is established (for at least three months).

How Fast (or Slowly) Should I Progress With Resistance Training?

In general, progression in repetitions or resistance level can occur every one to three weeks for healthy individuals under the age of 50 to 60. That progression should be slower for older or more frail individuals—every two to four weeks for healthy, older adults, or slower if necessary. Progress should always be individualized and based on tolerance. In other words, go by how you feel.

The rate of progression generally recommended for resistance training is 2 to 10 percent. This percentage refers to the level of resistance or the number of repetitions (it is best not to increase both at the same time). Smaller increases (2 to 5 percent) apply more to exercises that use smaller muscle groups and single joints (i.e., leg extensions, leg curls, bicep curls, tricep extensions). Larger increases (5 to 10 percent) apply more to exercises using larger muscle groups and multiple joints (i.e., squats, leg presses, lat pull downs, chest presses). When you can perform one to two additional repetitions fairly easily at your current level of intensity for one to two consecutive training sessions, chances are you can add a few more repetitions or a little more resistance.

> *Note:* To help you track your resistance training program, make copies of the resistance training log in Appendix N. List the exercises you are doing, and use the position/comments box to give yourself technique, safety, or personal reminders. Record the date, load, reps, and RPE. If you are doing multiple sets, you can divide the square for reps with a diagonal line and record number of sets. Documenting your resistance training workouts increases your level of safety, awareness, and motivation. Even if you are not inclined to do paperwork, *try it*.

Resistance Training With Disabilities and Chronic Diseases

Considering the fact that 88 percent of people over the age of 65 have one or more chronic diseases, specific recommendations for safe, effective exercise are essential. However, the *basic* physical needs of individuals who have one or more of the conditions listed in the following pages are the same as for anyone else (i.e., aerobic fitness, muscular strength/endurance, and flexibility).

Using resistance training to enhance muscular strength/endurance would fit into nearly any program. However, some modifications to guidelines should be made for certain conditions, and, of course, unique circumstances may be present that make the guidelines difficult to apply to your situation. In general, however, in the presence of a disease or disability, the priority with exercise is to:

• First restore or improve functional capabilities (Being able to perform activities of daily living with less pain and fatigue is of utmost importance.)

• Improve fitness

Be sure to consult your physician before beginning an exercise program, including resistance training. Follow the advice of your physician. You may also want to consult other health professionals or exercise specialists who know these clinical areas. It is important to approach exercise safely and not create more damage.

Follow the guidelines for those with disabilities and chronic diseases (Table 2-3) when applicable, but be sure to consult the information specific to individual conditions that follows. These guidelines are almost the same as those previously outlined for older or more frail individuals, with a little more caution advised.

The protective effect of exercise appears to increase with age.

Guidelines for Those With Disabilities and Chronic Diseases

Specific guidelines for those with disabilities and chronic diseases are not well established and will vary greatly. Please review the appropriate items in the next section of this chapter for more information. Consult with your physician and work with a knowledgeable exercise professional if possible, at least to get started. The following are general guidelines only—modify as necessary.

How many? Eight to ten exercises using all major muscle groups (arms, chest, abdomen, back, hips, and legs).

How much? One set of up to 10 to 15 repetitions of each exercise, or as tolerated (unless otherwise advised).

How often? Two to three times per week on nonconsecutive days (unless otherwise advised).

How hard? Intensity should be low (RPE 11 to 13, fairly light to somewhat hard). Progress slowly to allow time for adaptation. Sometimes, performing the motion with no added resistance is appropriate. If tolerated well, resistance training can usually be safely performed to muscle fatigue (with the exception of some neuromuscular diseases, as described in the next section of this chapter).

Table 2-3. Guidelines for those with disabilities and chronic diseases

Specific Resistance Training Guidelines for Disabilities and Chronic Diseases

This section is not light reading. The following information tends to be more technical and comprehensive than the previous sections. It is intended for anyone who wants or needs more detail in specific areas, either because they have or are associated with someone who has a particular medical condition. However, this information should not be regarded as a complete guide. It goes beyond the scope of this book to include extensive information for every disease. Rather, to the greatest extent possible (and feasible), this section includes the most pertinent points as identified by the author. If none of these conditions apply to you or interest you specifically, consider skipping or merely skimming over this section.

For many of the disabilities and chronic diseases discussed in the following pages, we don't have hard and fast recommendations for exercise. We are still learning and researching these areas. However, these guidelines are based on experience of professionals in the field and existing studies. *All guidelines are suggestions that may need modification based on tolerance and special needs.*

Also, keep in mind that these guidelines are primarily, but not exclusively, *resistance training* guidelines, meant to be only a part of a comprehensive fitness program that includes aerobic and flexibility exercises. Remember the tripod that was discussed in Chapter 1 (described in more detail in Appendix A).

In some instances, more than one health condition may be present. Use the guidelines common to *all* conditions. The following disabilities and chronic diseases are addressed in this section:

- ALS (Lou Gehrig's disease)
- Alzheimer's disease
- Arthritis
- Asthma
- Cancer
- Chronic fatigue syndrome
- Chronic obstructive pulmonary disease
- Chronic restrictive pulmonary disease
- Coronary heart disease
- Developmental disabilities
- Diabetes
- Epilepsy
- Fibromyalgia
- Frailty
- Hypertension (High blood pressure)
- Lower back pain syndrome
- Multiple sclerosis
- Muscular dystrophy
- Neuromuscular diseases
- Osteoporosis
- Overweight/obesity
- Parkinson's disease
- Peripheral arterial disease
- Physical disabilities
- Postpolio syndrome
- Stroke

ALS (Lou Gehrig's Disease) See Neuromuscular Diseases

Alzheimer's Disease See Neuromuscular Diseases

Arthritis

Resistance training is effective for people with the two most common forms of arthritis—*rheumatoid arthritis* (RA) and *osteoarthritis* (OA). (Weight loss can also significantly improve the symptoms associated with osteoarthritis. Refer to Overweight/Obesity later in this chapter. A weight loss of only five pounds can result in a decrease of 25 to 125 pounds of load on a joint.) Resistance training helps counteract pain, muscle weakness, mobility limitations, disability, and joint instability. *Resistance training does not make arthritis go away, nor does it make it worse.* Expect some discomfort, but do not do activities that increase joint pain. Adhere to the following guidelines:

Resistance training does not make arthritis go away, nor does it make it worse.

- Start with just squeezing the muscles individually (i.e., isometric contraction) and holding for 5 to 10 seconds, continuing to breathe as you do so. Squeezing prevents joints from having to flex or extend. Include all the major muscle groups.

- Strengthen painful joints in a similar fashion at angles (i.e., 45 degrees, 90 degrees). In other words, move joints through a full range of motion, pausing at different angles and squeezing muscles for 5 to 10 seconds. This action strengthens muscles throughout the range of motion but may be better tolerated than when moved continuously against resistance (such as when using an elastic band).

- Perform resistance training (when joints allow) through the full range of motion. Start with only two to three reps and build up gradually to 10 to 12 reps.

- Avoid or reduce resistance training during arthritis flare-ups, especially when accompanied by fever or extreme fatigue.

- Move all joints and major muscle groups through their full range of motion *every day* to maintain joint mobility, even on days of flare-ups when no other exercise is performed.

- Avoid vigorous, highly repetitive, or high-impact exercise.

- Avoid morning exercise if you experience prolonged muscle and joint stiffness after rising.

- Tie a knot at the ends of elastic bands if gripping is an issue. As an alternative, try light hand or wrist weights.

- Perform resistance training exercises in water, which results in significant muscle strength improvement and may be better tolerated than exercise on land.

- Stay informed regarding your condition. In the case of rheumatoid arthritis, an added risk of osteoporosis, heart and lung involvement, and cervical instability is present. Additionally, steroid use may lead to increased muscle weakness and bone loss, among other side effects.

- Consult an exercise professional. Existing or potential deformities may make some exercises awkward or dangerous for people with osteoarthritis or, especially, rheumatoid arthritis.

Asthma

Resistance training usually does not trigger asthma symptoms often seen with aerobic activities because it is not continuous in nature. When exercise-induced asthma is well controlled, or asthma is mild, follow the age-appropriate Guidelines for Healthy Adults (Table 2-1). For moderate/severe asthma, follow the General Guidelines for Those With Disabilities and Chronic Diseases (Table 2-3) outlined at the beginning of this section. In most cases, practicing special breathing techniques (e.g., pursed-lips breathing) can help reduce the sensation of breathlessness (refer to Appendix E).

Cancer

Individualized mild- to moderate-intensity exercise during cancer treatment and beyond can improve physical function (aerobic capacity, muscular strength, flexibility, and body composition). It can also help combat symptoms of treatment (nausea, fatigue, weight change, poor sleep) and the emotional impact of treatment (depression, anxiety, low self-esteem, loss of control). Little research is available to provide clear exercise guidelines for those with cancer, and most existing studies have focused on cancer survivors or those with early-stage disease and a good prognosis. However, what information does exist supports the benefit of exercise for cancer survivors as well as for many going through treatment (postsurgery, chemotherapy, or radiation), as long as exercise is individualized based on unique disease- and treatment-related limitations.

Exercise can reduce the intensity of fatigue during cancer treatment by 15 to 35 percent and helps avoid the deconditioning that accompanies too much rest.

Fatigue is the most common symptom experienced during cancer treatment, occurring in an estimated 70 to 95 percent of patients, and can last months or even years. Though rest is an approach often used to combat fatigue, exercise can reduce the intensity of fatigue by 15 to 35 percent and helps avoid the deconditioning that accompanies too much rest. Though exercise may seem like the last thing you want to do when fatigued, it appears that doing even very little may help. Many of the concerns relating exercise to cancer, including the unwillingness or inability to tolerate exercise, are being dispelled. In most cases, it seems safe, effective, and feasible. It should be approached as a quality of life, rather than a curative intervention.

In the latest publications, resistance training is emerging as a recommended part of the guidelines for exercise, combined with some form of aerobic exercise such as walking or stationary cycling. Radiation and chemotherapy disturb muscle integrity and cause muscle tissue loss, and can result in extreme muscle weakness, fatigue, muscle imbalances, and decreased range of motion. Physical inactivity exacerbates this condition. These symptoms may improve significantly with exercise. Until further guidelines are available, follow the General Guidelines for Those With Disabilities and Chronic Diseases (Table 2-3), keeping in mind the following:

- Resistance training should be started with just range of motion and should be progressed *gradually* to using light weight as tolerated.

- Weight machines often have loads too heavy to start with—light hand weights (one to three pounds), elastic bands, balls, or tubing may be more appropriate.

- Repetitions may be only three to five to start with, increasing gradually to 10 to 12.

- *Gradual* progression is essential. Make adjustments according to current treatment and state of the disease.

- High-intensity exercise should be avoided during cancer treatment, although this kind of exercise seems safe for most cancer survivors.

- Flexibility exercises (i.e., stretching) should be attempted even on "down days" during periods of chemotherapy treatment.

- Special precautions or complications that would affect choice or intensity of exercise include low blood counts (see your doctor), fever, dizziness, severe weight loss, shortness of breath, bone pain, nausea, dehydration, and extreme fatigue. In the event that you experience any of these symptoms, stop or reduce exercise intensity (i.e., lighter loads, shorter duration, or no added resistance). Discuss any concerns with your physician. Exercising in short, intermittent sessions throughout the day may be best tolerated.

- Activities that increase risk (e.g., having physical contact or doing high-impact activities when experiencing bone pain or low platelet counts, swimming when neutrophil counts are low due to risk of bacterial infection, participating in activities that require coordination or balance when dizzy) should be avoided. Watch for signs of swelling, particularly lymphydema, which can sometimes occur after having breast cancer surgery. Tracking arm circumference measurements can be helpful to monitor this condition.

- If a medicine port has been placed, exercises should be monitored closely so as not to interfere with the port location.

- Be mindful of pain from surgical scarring. Reduce range of motion.

- Given the predictable ups and downs during and following cancer treatment, progression in your exercise may be often interrupted. Be patient and flexible. Enlist the help of an exercise or health professional.

Chronic Fatigue Syndrome (CFS)

Unfortunately, very little is known about the origins and treatment of this condition. Exercise among people who suffer from CFS has often been accompanied by increased fatigue and worsening symptoms. However, this side-effect seems to be true only initially or when accompanied by an increase in the activities of daily living. An overall improvement in symptoms has been reported when accompanied by exercise.

Practicing standard exercise techniques does not successfully return those with CFS to a normal, healthy status, and it can lead to exacerbation. Focus on reducing symptoms, preventing further deconditioning, preserving the ability to perform activities of daily living, and avoiding relapse. Adhere to the following guidelines:

- All exercise should range from very light to light intensity on the RPE scale. Progress should be *extremely* gradual. Avoid the tendency to overdo exercise or daily activities when feeling good.

- Stretching should be done daily, particularly earlier in the day. Neck stretches can help relieve headaches.

- Try performing resistance training and low-level aerobic exercise on alternate days rather than on the same day.

- Initially, no added resistance should be used for strengthening. Rather, active motion using just your own body weight against gravity is appropriate to start.

- Consider delaying the use of added resistance (i.e., elastic bands, hand weights, machines) until three sets of 15 repetitions can be done with no added resistance (i.e., by just going through the motions). The three sets could be split throughout the day if better tolerated.

- Strengthening exercises should first focus on trunk stability, followed by arm and leg strengthening.

- Specifically, resistance training should seek to preserve levels of strength needed to perform activities of daily living while attempting to avoid muscle soreness.

Chronic Obstructive Pulmonary Disease (COPD)

COPD primarily includes emphysema and chronic bronchitis. Individuals with COPD have significant muscle weakness and loss of muscle mass, in part due to deconditioning, possible steroid use, and the disease itself. People with this disease can experience a 20 to 30 percent loss of strength, particularly in the quadriceps (front of thigh), as well as significantly less mechanical efficiency with leg exercises (about 15 percent) compared to healthy people (about 25 percent). Arm mechanical efficiency seems to be well preserved in those with COPD and is similar to healthy people. Resistance training is recommended for those with COPD, though not much research exists to provide guidelines. Until such recommendations exist, follow the General Guidelines for Those With Disabilities and Chronic Diseases (Table 2-3). Also note the following:

- Pursed-lips breathing should be coordinated with resistance exercise movements to help reduce shortness of breath, inhaling to the count of two and exhaling to the count of four. For guidance on breathing techniques, see Appendix E. Also refer to Breathlessness Scale in Appendix D.

- Always exhale on the effort, completing one to two repetitions per exhale. *Always pause to inhale.*

- Late morning to early afternoon is a good time of day to exercise for those with COPD.

- Exercising within one to two hours of taking routine inhaled medications will help your breathing during exercise.

- Avoid exercising outdoors when temperature and humidity are high.

- Modify your program on bad breathing days, shortening your exercise sessions based on your tolerance. This stipulation could mean exercising from as little as 30 seconds to three minutes at a time. On bad breathing days, resistance train with little to no added resistance (i.e., just go through the motions).

Chronic Restrictive Pulmonary Disease (CRPD)

CRPD includes interstitial lung diseases such as pulmonary fibrosis and sarcoidosis, kyphoscoliosis, and, in some cases, severe obesity. Similar to COPD, not much exists in the way of research to recommend guidelines. Follow the General Guidelines for Those With Disabilities and Chronic Diseases (Table 2-3). Coordinating resistance exercises with pursed-lips breathing is helpful. However, prolonging your exhalation as described for COPD (at least twice as long as the inhalation) is not necessary (for further guidelines on breathing techniques, see Appendix E). Similar to those with COPD, late morning or early afternoon is a good time of day to exercise. Also, try to avoid exercising outdoors when the temperature and humidity are high. Monitor breathlessness by referring to the scale in Appendix D.

Coronary Heart Disease (CHD)

Light to moderate intensity resistance training (even high intensity in some cases) has been shown to be safe, effective, and very important in an exercise program for most people with cardiac disease. In fact, resistance training is proving to be safe when combined with aerobic programs fairly early in cardiac rehabilitation. Compared with aerobic exercise at similar levels, resistance training generally doesn't result in chest pain (angina) or worrisome heart rhythm changes. Blood pressure does increase, but is "clinically acceptable" when intensity and heart rate are moderate. In fact, the higher blood pressure actually seems to be beneficial, as the heart muscle itself receives more blood between beats. Resistance training ultimately helps to reduce the load on the heart during activities of daily living, and it helps to reduce body fat and increase muscle mass. The increase in muscle mass can also improve aerobic capacity. The following information is based on ACSM/AACVPR guidelines. (Also be sure to follow the guidelines in Table 2-3.)

Resistance training *is* safe in the event of:

- Post-heart attack
- Post-open heart surgery (including bypass, valve repair, and congenital defect repairs)

- Post-stent/angioplasty
- Stable angina (chest pain associated with physical or mental stress)
- Uncomplicated atrial fibrillation
- Pacemakers (including AICD)
- Mild/moderate valve disease
- Stable congestive heart failure
- Post-cardiac transplant

Resistance training is *not* safe in the event of:

- Unstable angina (chest pain not associated with physical or mental stress, that is, at rest)
- Some uncontrolled heart rhythm disturbances
- Uncontrolled high blood pressure (systolic ≥ 160 mmHg, diastolic ≥ 105 mmHg)
- Unstable and symptomatic congestive heart failure
- Certain significant valve diseases
- Poor function of the left ventricle

> Always talk to your cardiologist to see if you are a candidate for safe resistance training with your specific cardiac diagnosis. Moderate- to high-risk patients are strongly encouraged to attend cardiac rehabilitation for supervision. At the very least, all cardiac patients should be given exercise guidelines by their doctor. Consulting further with a trained health professional is highly recommended.

How soon is it safe to resistance train? The following time-course guidelines are general and will vary with healing rates and possible complications. Also follow the General Guidelines for Those With Disabilities and Chronic Diseases (Table 2-3).

- *Heart attack:* Low-level resistance training (RPE 11) with light elastic bands or hand weights (one to two pounds) can be initiated by three weeks after an uncomplicated heart attack. Regular free weights or machines can typically be used at four to six weeks. Programs should also include consistent supervised aerobic exercise.

- *Bypass surgery:* Begin upper body range of motion only activities (24 to 48 hours after surgery) and very light resistance (one to two pounds) during convalescence. Moderate to heavy resistance training (RPE 13 to 15) should not be initiated until healing of sternum (breastbone) is complete (about three months postsurgery) and should be checked by doctor for stability.

- *Angioplasty or stent:* If stable, resistance training can be initiated three weeks postprocedure. May benefit by first participating for two weeks in a consistent supervised aerobic program such as cardiac rehabilitation.

- *Congestive/chronic heart failure (CHF):* Sixty-eight percent of patients with CHF have severe muscle wasting, in part because of the deconditioning from physical inactivity. Some skepticism exists about whether resistance training for those with CHF would make their condition worse. However, it is now generally recognized as safe for stable CHF conditions. In fact, when severe heart rhythm disturbances have been ruled out and drug therapy has been well tolerated over time, resistance training has been shown to improve muscular strength, muscle function, muscle metabolism, and blood flow. Improved blood vessel function leads to favorable changes in muscle fiber types and has positive effects on heart function. These changes can reduce the fatigue, shortness of breath and activity intolerance suffered by those with CHF. It has been recommended that resistance training focus more on small muscle groups and be reduced to one to two times per week.

- *Heart transplant:* Resistance training can and should be safely implemented two months posttransplant. Large strength increases of 40 to 50 percent are seen in exercise studies on heart transplant and resistance training. A significant loss in fat-free mass occurs in the first two months posttransplant. Resistance training programs of only seven weeks can restore muscle mass to pre-transplant levels, and programs of six months can result in increases of muscle mass beyond pre-transplant levels. Further, resistance training helps restore the bone mineral density lost by steroid use, even as steroid use continues posttransplant.

- *Post-heart transplant:* Perform resistance training two days per week, doing 12 to 15 repetitions. Include seven to eight exercises, using all major muscle groups. Include a low back extension exercise, as studies show a 10 to 20 percent loss of bone mineral density in the low back spine in only two months as a result of heavy steroid use. For safety, use minimal load on spine and perform low back extension only one day per week. With your physician's permission, low intensity resistance training can also be offered to those awaiting transplant.

Developmental Disabilities (DD)

Resistance training is safe, effective, and important for individuals with mental retardation and other developmental disabilities. However, initially those with DD require a great deal of supervision and clear feedback from an exercise or health specialist familiar with exercise technique. Use simple instructions and stress frequent safety guidelines. Diagrams and renaming exercises to describe the action may help in teaching the exercises. *Precaution: Approximately 17 percent of all individuals with Down syndrome have neck instability. When this condition is present, exercises that may strain the neck should be avoided.* In the absence of other medical conditions, those with DD can follow the age-appropriate Guidelines for Healthy Adults (Table 2-1). Otherwise, follow the General Guidelines for Those With Disabilities and Chronic Diseases (Table 2-3).

Diabetes

Though much more research is needed, early studies show resistance training is safe and beneficial for those with *controlled* diabetes (both Type I and II), especially when combined with aerobic exercise. Improvements are seen in insulin sensitivity and blood sugar uptake, in part by increasing muscle mass. This exercise also assists with weight loss, often needed for those with Type II diabetes. Follow the General Guidelines for Those With Disabilities and Chronic Diseases (Table 2-3) and the following specific recommendations:

- Monitor and maintain proper glucose levels and adjust insulin doses (if applicable).
- For Type I diabetes and Type II diabetes requiring use of insulin or oral hypoglycemic medications, avoid exercise when blood glucose is over 250 mg/dl with ketosis, and over 300 mg/dl without ketosis.
- Be sure blood glucose is at least 80 to 100 mg/dl to avoid hypoglycemia (low blood sugar). If low, eat a high quality snack before exercise.
- Avoid exercising late in the evening, as it increases the risk of nighttime low blood sugar.
- Wear proper footwear and regularly check feet for cracks, sores, or red areas.
- Keep hydrated.
- Maintain normal breathing throughout range of motion.
- Avoid marked increases in blood pressure by steering clear of intense, jarring, or straining-type activities (such as heavy resistance training), and also excessive gripping. This practice is especially important in those with kidney disease and advanced retinopathy.
- Avoid exercise if you have active retinal hemorrhage or have had recent treatment for retinopathy.

Epilepsy See Neuromuscular Diseases

Fibromyalgia

Fibromyalgia is usually considered a type of arthritis, but it is a noninflammatory, soft-tissue rheumatism rather than a joint disease. It can involve any number of 18 standard trigger points. People diagnosed with fibromyalgia have tenderness in at least 11 of the 18 trigger points for three months or longer. Very little research exists in the use of resistance training in people with fibromyalgia, but limited evidence shows a moderate to strong effectiveness. Though symptoms may initially worsen, tolerance tends to improve as the exercise program continues. Avoid morning exercise when discomfort levels may be higher.

Follow the previous guidelines for Arthritis. Aquatic resistance training may also be a well-tolerated option for people with fibromyalgia.

Frailty

Older adults are vulnerable to becoming frail. Frailty results from the loss of physical function. Once frailty sets in, it is difficult to reverse. Women are at much greater risk for frailty than men. They suffer losses of muscle strength and mass, as well as bone density, starting at an earlier age and a faster rate compared to men. Because of this factor, women are at higher risk for falling and sustaining fractures. On average, muscle strength is lost at about 1 to 2 percent per year after the age of 30. Between 50 and 70 years of age, strength declines as much as 30 percent, with even larger decreases after the age of 80. This decrease is due to a loss in the size and number of muscle fibers.

Women are at much greater risk for frailty than are men.

The specific physical fitness components that provide physical function are muscle strength, muscle endurance, balance, and flexibility. Resistance training improves the levels of each of these components. However, aerobic exercise, balance training, and flexibility training do *not* improve muscle mass or strength. They cannot be a substitute for resistance training. Resistance training is the most effective way to reduce loss of muscle mass associated with aging, estimated to be a 20 to 50 percent loss for both men and women over the adult life span. Though the amount of muscle mass that can be gained with resistance training doesn't seem dramatic (i.e., an average of a two-pound increase), resistance training stops the dramatic loss of significant amounts of muscle mass seen in those who are not resistance training.

As discussed in the section Overweight/Obesity, the increased strength from resistance training can improve your ability to walk at faster speeds, walk for longer distances, and perform more activities of daily living. This kind of exercise will not only improve aerobic fitness and balance, but it will help to reduce fat weight that often accompanies aging. More specifically, resistance training can significantly reduce the amount of abdominal fat that has a tendency to accumulate with age, especially in postmenopausal women. This benefit can occur even in the absence of fat weight changes in other areas of the body. A decrease in abdominal fat not only reduces waistline girth (having cosmetic appeal to most people), but, more importantly, it also reduces the risk of heart disease and diabetic/metabolic disorders associated with abdominal obesity. *Risk increases with abdominal girth measures of over 40 inches for men and 35 inches for women.*

For healthy older adults to safely resistance train, follow the Guidelines for Healthy Adults 50-60+ Years of Age or More Frail Individuals (Table 2-2). If medical conditions are present, follow the General Guidelines for Those With Disabilities and Chronic Diseases (Table 2-3). Watch for dizziness and loss of balance. Avoid hyperextension of the neck and back. Watch for exacerbation of other diseases/medical conditions.

Hypertension (High blood pressure)

In the past, resistance training for those with hypertension was discouraged because of concerns regarding impact on the heart and brain. It has since been shown to be quite safe. However, resistance training has not been consistently shown to *lower* blood pressure (with the exception of lowered blood pressures in response to an endurance method called circuit weight training). Therefore, it is not recommended as a primary activity, rather, as a part of a *well-rounded* program including aerobic exercise. Higher-load resistance training should be avoided, particularly in those whose blood pressure is 180/110 mmHg or more. Individuals without cardiac disease can follow the age-appropriate Guidelines for Healthy Adults (Table 2-1). For individuals with hypertension and cardiac disease, or those without cardiac disease that want a more conservative approach, follow the General Guidelines for Those With Disabilities and Chronic Disease (Table 2-3). Avoid straining and holding your breath while exerting against resistance.

Lower Back Pain Syndrome (LBP)

Lower back pain is one of the most commonly experienced and most expensive health problems in the world. It is a condition that ends up merely managed rather than cured. Lifetime prevalence is almost 60 to 70 percent, and the chances that back pain will reoccur within a year are 50 percent. Very few low back injuries occur from a single, specific event—usually, they happen as a result of stresses on the tissues over time. Part of what makes this condition difficult to manage is that letting "pain be your guide" doesn't always work very well. Pain isn't always related to injury, and it can continue long after an injury heals. In other words, pain and injury (hurt and harm) are not one and the same when associated with low back pain. Further, though millions seek traditional health care for diagnosis and treatment, doctors can reportedly verify a diagnosis less than 5 percent of the time. Similar to the cause of injury, the cause of the pain isn't usually a result of any one specific issue. Rather, an injury sensitizes all of the surrounding tissues. Hence, back pain is often referred to as *nonspecific*.

> When it comes to back pain, letting "pain be your guide" doesn't always work very well.

The guidelines for back pain promote self-management and exercise. Although avoiding physical activity with sudden, acute pain where pain and injury are related is appropriate for the short-term, it is not constructive for the long-term. The following guidelines help to determine whether your back pain is acute (short-term) or chronic (long-term):

• *Acute LBP* is when symptoms last less than 6 to 12 weeks. Returning to early normal activity is the primary goal and should be limited by time, not pain. Recovery should happen within days or weeks, regardless of how it is managed. Specific exercises have not been shown to be particularly useful. Rather, a return to normal activities (after one to two days of rest) can best ensure a faster recovery from symptoms. Actual structured exercise should be started within the first two weeks of acute LBP. Choose exercises that minimize the load on the back. Do not do high-impact exercises such as running. Choose postures that are best tolerated (i.e., standing versus sitting). Feel free to do exercises that allow your best effort. Wait two weeks to begin trunk and hip exercises, and, then, do so at a very low intensity and with slow progression (refer to the sections on back exercises in Chapters 4 and 5). Maintain the strength of the back muscles with the back extension exercise (Figures 4-18 and 4-19) performed at a low resistance and higher repetitions (12 to 15 repetitions, one to two times per week).

- *Chronic LBP* is defined as having symptoms persisting beyond 12 weeks. It does seem that exercise and activity are helpful, but mostly because exercise helps to reduce the perception and fear of pain and to improve a sense of well-being. While many specific regimens are designed for back care, it has been said that the most effective exercise or activity regimen is the one the individual will actually perform.

Your back is feeling good and you want to keep it that way? Contrary to popular belief, trunk (torso) strength and flexibility are *not* strong predictors of LBP or disability. Rather, poor general health is the strongest predictor for new LBP, and a previous history of LBP is one of the most reliable predictors of recurrent LBP. Poor lumbar (low back) muscle strength is often a predictor of back injury. Because of the initial weakness in this muscle group in most people, 12 to 15 repetitions done one to two times per week at a low intensity is recommended (Chapter 4). Use proper technique with resistance training and maintain excellent posture at all times (Figures 3-1 and 3-2), maintaining the natural curves of the spine, and develop good core strength (abdominal/back muscles) in a well-rounded program. These guidelines all minimize the risk of acute back injury. Refer to back strengthening exercises (Chapter 4) and stretches (Chapter 5).

Multiple Sclerosis See Neuromuscular Diseases

Muscular Dystrophy See Neuromuscular Diseases

Neuromuscular Diseases

Progressive neuromuscular diseases mean the condition will worsen over time. The following disorders are progressive (*nonprogressive* disorders are listed under Physical Disabilities later in this section). Progressive disorders require closer monitoring to be sure resistance training is not causing an exacerbation (worsening). When muscle soreness occurs in persons with a progressive neuromuscular disorder, it may mean overload, or overwork weakness. Though this fact is not yet well established by research, overloading when a neuromuscular disease is present could result in permanent strength loss. Until more is known, it is important to be extremely cautious. Get clear and specific exercise recommendations from your physician. In general, resistance training for those with a neuromuscular disease is most beneficial if:

- The degree of weakness isn't severe (≤ 30 percent functional muscle mass affected)
- Progression of the disease is slow
- Rate of increasing exercise intensity is slow and supervised
- Activities of daily living are wisely paced

ALS (Lou Gehrig's Disease): ALS is the most common of the neuromuscular diseases. It results in muscular weakness and can be rapidly progressive. Exercise is most beneficial in early stages and in those with slow progression. Any exercise program will need to be readjusted as function declines. Use no added resistance with resistance training—range of motion only. Avoid excessive fatigue.

Alzheimer's Disease: Ten percent of people living in the community (i.e., not institutionalized) over the age of 65 and fully 40 percent of those age 85 and older have Alzheimer's disease. Some research shows that exercise can improve brain resiliency and efficiency, the ability to learn, and the ability to communicate in individuals with Alzheimer's disease. Also, some indication is present that increased physical activity will reduce the risk of Alzheimer's. Exercise with a partner, a group, or some form of supervision is recommended. Focus on range of motion and strength. Try exercising in the morning when agitation levels are often lower or in intermittent bouts.

Epilepsy: When seizures are controlled, individuals with epilepsy have no restrictions with resistance training. The age-appropriate Guidelines for Healthy Adults (Table 2-1) can be followed if younger than 50- to 60-years-old and no other conditions are present, though it is a good idea to start with low resistance and high repetitions.

Multiple Sclerosis (MS): Resistance training appears safe and effective for those with MS. Exercise has no effect on the progression of MS but can improve fitness and function. Factors that may affect exercise tolerance are fatigue, balance issues, heat intolerance, spasticity, reduced sensation, numbness, tingling, or partial/total paralysis (more common in lower extremities). Start with low level of resistance and perform resistance training on nonaerobic exercise days. Exercising in the pool may help control heat-related intolerance. Exacerbations may occur frequently or infrequently, depending on the degree of involvement. After an exacerbation, restart at a lower level of resistance than used before the exacerbation.

Muscular Dystrophy (MD): Studies provide no evidence that exercise results in a more rapid loss of strength. About half of those in these studies that participate in moderate resistance training and stretching experience mild improvements in strength. Muscles with mild to moderate weakness are the most likely to respond favorably. Low resistance should be used initially and increased gradually as tolerated over weeks to months. When muscles become too weak, the goal becomes moving through available range of motion and preventing contractures. Stretching should be done daily. Be aware of possible cardiac involvement or low bone mass, and check special recommendations in this section for those conditions.

Parkinson's Disease: Resistance training appears to be effective in combating the effects of Parkinson's, though few studies have included aerobic and strengthening exercise. Further, considerable variability in symptoms makes it difficult to assess the effectiveness of exercise interventions. Follow the General Guidelines for Those With Disabilities and Chronic Diseases (Table 2-3) as long as ability allows. Resistance training, if tolerated, may be safer on machines than using bands or free weights. Wrist and ankle weights may also be a safe option. Exercise should target motor control problems such as range of motion/flexibility, balance, gait, mobility, and coordination exercises. Supervised exercise or exercising with a partner is a good idea. Make sure you have a railing, chair, or some support nearby, and avoid complex movements.

Postpolio Syndrome (PPS): PPS can occur several decades after the onset of polio and affects about 25 percent of those who contracted the polio virus in the 1950s to 1960s. The extent of damage varies considerably. Symptoms include fatigue, joint/muscle pain, progressive muscle weakness (in polio-damaged muscles as well as undamaged muscles), respiratory problems, and cold intolerance. Many individuals deal with spasms, pain, weakness, and full or partial loss of sensation. Few studies exist on resistance training with PPS, but most experts agree that not including resistance training will lead to loss of function. The significantly reduced leg strength associated with PPS can be improved with resistance training, using the following guidelines:

- Avoid muscle fatigue. Begin with minimal resistance and progress slowly.

- Take frequent rest breaks during exercise sessions. You may want to exercise different muscles on alternate days (i.e., upper body one day, lower body the next).

- Use your "best" muscles. In other words, exercise the muscles that are least affected. Be more protective of the muscles that have the most impairment.

- Stop resistance training and switch to aerobic and flexibility exercises if muscles become fatigued or sore. Overestimating maximal effort may accelerate motor unit loss. Loss of strength due to excessive overload may be permanent. Supervision by a trained health professional is recommended for at least two months when an exercise program is initiated. Frequent ongoing follow-up is advised.

- Exercise is best tolerated in the morning at low-stress times. Exercising in a warm pool may be a great option for those with PPS.

Osteoporosis

Osteoporosis is diagnosed when approximately 25 percent bone reduction exists. Bone health may be 60 to 80 percent genetic—80 percent of those with osteoporosis are women, especially those who are slender, white, and with fair-complexion. Smoking, as well as excessive caffeine and alcohol intake, further increases the risk of osteoporosis. Yet another important contributing factor that occurs long before the actual onset of osteoporosis is the amount of bone mineral density present when a young adult reaches peak bone mass. This factor calls for early attention to calcium intake and physical activity levels during the preteen/teenage years.

Studies have shown that bone density can increase with resistance training, though the response is relatively small (2 to 3 percent) and relatively slow (four to six months minimum, with optimal results after one year of training). Not surprisingly, young bone seems more responsive than older bone. However, the most effective resistance training programs have been the ones that are high intensity (75 to 85 percent of maximum strength), lower repetition, and high impact (at least three times your body weight). The lumbar (low back) forces during brisk walking are about one times body weight, while the forces during running are estimated to be about 1.75 to 2 times body weight. The forces during resistance training in the standing position have been estimated to equal up to five to six times body weight. Therefore, resistance training, particularly in the standing position, seems to be more effective at increasing bone mineral density than aerobic training (Graves & Franklin, eds., 2001). However, given the fact that those who suffer most from osteoporosis tend to be older individuals, often frail and susceptible to fracture, high intensity resistance training, particularly over the period of a year, may not be a safe approach, especially without trained supervision.

Though lower intensity resistance training and weight-bearing aerobic exercise may not be the most effective way to *increase* bone mineral density, doing those kinds of exercises may *reduce* further loss of bone mass. Particularly if the actual goal is to reduce the risk of falling, thereby reducing the risk of fracture, it is probably *more* important to focus on using resistance training to improve muscular strength rather than to be focused on increasing bone mineral density. Even without increases in bone mineral density, improving muscular strength in the legs can reduce the risk of falls. Muscle, unlike bone, responds readily to training. Incorporating a more general, well-rounded moderate intensity resistance training program reduces the risk of becoming injured from a high intensity program, and also helps reduce the risk of falling.

Certain resistance training exercises are effective in impacting bone density by involving muscles that "pull" directly at the locations of fracture risk (e.g., hip, spine, forearm/wrist). This type of movement has the potential to stimulate bone to increase in density. It may also be beneficial to vary the exercises used and add exercises that safely allow greater loads.

You can lose bone at a faster rate by being physically inactive, than you can gain bone by being active.
—Barbara Drinkwater, Ph.D.

In conclusion, based on available research, the following recommendations are optimum resistance training guidelines for bone health. Start with one set of 10 to 15 repetitions (fewer if necessary). If not yet osteoporotic (or if given medical clearance), *gradually* increase to three sets of 8 to 12 repetitions three times per week for a minimum of one year at moderate to high intensity. Choose 6 to 12 of the specific exercises for osteoporosis in Chapter 4 (Target Strengthening for Osteoporosis). Note: To reduce the risk of vertebral fractures in those who already have osteoporosis, avoid forward flexion and twisting of the spine, especially when combined with stooping. Always maintain the natural curves of the spine and bend from the hips, *not* the middle of the back. Avoid quick, jarring movements, particularly when combined with a twisting motion. If back pain limits the ability to do weight-bearing exercise, do chair or water exercise. Be sure to seek the advice of a physician before beginning a program.

Overweight/Obesity

The prevalence of obesity has dramatically increased in the past decade and is associated with many health conditions. Sixty-five percent of the adult U.S. population is considered to be overweight (defined as having a Body Mass Index (BMI) of > 25), and 30 percent of the adult U.S. population is considered to be obese (BMI > 30). (To identify your BMI, consult the table in Appendix J). Though most studies have evaluated the effect of aerobic training on weight loss, resistance training is a potentially important component of an overall program for body weight and fat loss. This fact is primarily because resistance training can preserve and even increase muscle mass. Average increases with resistance training are two to five pounds, and a five-pound increase in muscle mass is associated with an increase of about a 50-calorie energy expenditure per day. (To estimate your daily energy expenditure both at rest and with activities, see Appendices H and I).

The popular hype publicizing resistance training as turning you into a "calorie-burning machine" is vastly overrated.

However, the popular hype publicizing resistance training as turning you into a "calorie-burning machine" is vastly overrated. Unfortunately, the studies do not show resistance training to be an added benefit when combined with dieting (calorie restriction) for weight loss when compared to endurance exercise alone or dieting only. Contrary to popular belief, resistance training does not seem to prevent the decline in resting energy expenditure that occurs with dieting. Therefore, resistance training cannot really be supported as a superior method of weight loss compared to other more commonly used methods.

Nonetheless, the value of resistance training in an overall program should not be underestimated, even when weight loss is the goal. The increased strength from resistance training can improve the ability to walk at faster speeds, walk for longer distances, and perform more activities of daily living. Further, just a one-pound weight loss results in a reduction in load of 5 to 10 pounds on the joints, which is important, especially when arthritis is present in addition to carrying extra weight.

Additionally, as previously discussed in the section on Frailty, resistance training can significantly reduce the amount of abdominal fat that has a tendency to accumulate with age, especially in postmenopausal women. Abdominal fat accumulation can occur even in the absence of fat weight changes in other areas of the body. Resistance training not only reduces abdominal girth, which has cosmetic appeal to most people, but, more importantly, it also reduces the risk of heart disease, diabetes and other health disorders that are associated with abdominal obesity. The level of risk increases when abdominal girth measures over 40 inches for men and 35 inches for women.

In conclusion, the most effective weight-loss regimen, based on the research so far, includes a combination of the following:

- Moderate intensity aerobic exercise—a minimum of 150 minutes per week (i.e., 30 minutes a day, five days a week). Ideally, progress to 200 to 300 minutes (2000-plus kcal) per week. Moderate levels of lifestyle physical activity may be included with structured exercise (use the Physical Activity Record in Appendix O to track weekly activity). Also refer to Appendix G for easy ways to become more physically active.

- Resistance training two to three times a week (use the Resistance Training Log in Appendix N to track the program)

- Reducing food intake (reduce by 500 to 1000 calories kcal a day, depending on overall intake and activity levels) and reducing dietary fat to less than 30 percent of total intake, with a goal of one to two pounds per week of weight loss. Use the Food Record in Appendix Q to document and track intake. Be sure you are eating at least 1200 kcal a day for adequate energy and proper nutrition.

- Identifying your readiness to change (Appendix K), establishing social support, recording goal setting/problem solving (Appendix L), and self-monitoring eating and exercise behaviors

A one-pound weight loss results in the reduction in load of 5 to 10 pounds on the joints.

Fortunately, ideal body weights do not need to be achieved to enjoy positive health benefits—even a 5 to 10 percent weight loss will significantly improve health, including blood pressure, blood lipids, and Type II diabetes risk. Be aware that the weight loss effect from exercise can be significantly influenced by genetic differences between individuals, so that not everyone responds to the same volume of exercise in the same way, even when intake is the same. Evidence also exists that exercise for weight loss is more effective for men than for women. Regardless of these differences, long-term weight loss has a poor success rate, especially in the absence of a regular exercise program, and overweight/obesity issues require lifelong management.

Parkinson's Disease See Neuromuscular Diseases

Peripheral Arterial Disease (PAD), Peripheral Vascular Occlusive Disease (PVOD), or Peripheral Vascular Disease (PVD)

PAD is caused by an occlusion of blood flow through the arteries of the legs and affects up to 20 percent of older adults. The resulting cramps occur in the thighs or calves, and, depending on the location of the blockage, sometimes begin in the buttocks. This intermittent lack of sufficient oxygen can result in actual changes in muscle fiber types in the calf (i.e., a decreased area of muscle fibers and a reduced number of aerobic endurance muscle fibers) leading to earlier muscle fatigue. Resistance training is helpful for those with PAD. The enhanced muscle mass encourages increased oxygen to the muscles. Recommended resistance exercises include calf raises, leg extensions, leg curls, and leg abductions/adductions. Use lighter loads and perform 10 to 20 repetitions to promote adequate blood flow during muscle contraction with less stress on the cardiovascular system. Regular stretching of these muscle groups also improves oxygen use and blood flow. Follow the General Guidelines for Those With Disabilities and Chronic Diseases (Table 2-3). Also consult Target Strengthening for Peripheral Arterial Disease in Chapter 4.

Women have been shown to have worse outcomes and to experience greater limitations than men with PAD. They experience intermittent pain sooner, begin walking shorter distances and at slower speeds, and see themselves as having less ability to successfully climb stairs compared to men. Women with PAD are less likely to be physically active overall and more likely to live dependent lifestyles compared to men.

However discouraging this news may seem if you are a woman with PAD, studies show that most of these differences are simply explained by lower fitness levels in women and the accompanying lower confidence compared to men. Therefore, exercise—aerobic and resistance training—is essential and can shift these differences seen between men and women. Regular walking is recommended, and those with PAD are encouraged to tolerate pain with walking as long as possible beyond the onset of pain (sometimes only one to two minutes) and at a relatively high intensity (see Rating of Claudication (PAD) Discomfort During Exercise Scale in Appendix D), allowing full recovery during rests. Intersperse walking with other nonweight-bearing activities, including upper body exercises, especially in the beginning.

Physical Disabilities

Persons with physical disabilities have an especially high risk of becoming dependent on others to meet basic activities of daily living. When combined with the high incidence of physical inactivity and poor health practices, individuals with physical disabilities often live close to the threshold of needing assistance. This risk increases with increasing age. Because of this factor, a high risk is present of overuse injuries and fatigue.

Resistance training has the potential to significantly improve function and quality of life. However, programs must be individually customized to allow those with physical disabilities to meet their unique demands of daily living, overcome physical barriers, and improve quality of life. The disabilities outlined previously in Neuromuscular Diseases can also be defined as *physical disabilities*, and are often progressive in nature. Other conditions, such as *cerebral palsy* and *spinal cord injury* are not progressive. Those with nonprogressive disorders can usually work at higher intensity levels than those with progressive disorders.

Many potential challenges have to be dealt with, including one-sided weakness, partial or complete paralysis, spasticity or the opposite (flaccid muscle tone), pressure sores, and contractures. The following list provides some guidance in considering a program. The resistance training program depends on what the physical disability is, the severity of the disability, overall health status, and related conditions.

- The lower the amount of functional muscle mass, the lower the training volume should be.

- Since spasticity (rigid muscle tone or tightness) is often present, flexibility exercises should always accompany resistance training. Use slow, controlled movements. It may not be possible to fully extend a severely spastic muscle. Resistance training may cause a temporary increase in spasticity on the affected or nonaffected side. This affect should disappear soon after a session is completed. Spastic muscles do not necessarily mean they are strong—strengthen them.

- Free weights, elastic bands, or machines can be used effectively if they are safe for the individual. However, the risk of dropping weights or snapping bands is present if loss of control happens.

- Free weights for persons with physical disabilities can be easily modified to resemble activities of daily living. However, they may be difficult and unsafe for those without good trunk stability and limitations in motor control and coordination.

- Use light resistance for at least the first month. Increase the load only if no soreness or fatigue is present.

- For those with extreme weakness, simply lifting limbs and the body against gravity without added resistance may be enough to start, possibly enlisting active assistance from a partner.

- Each individual needs to start by not doing much more than they are accustomed to on a daily basis. Those prone to seizures or fatigue should reduce training volume.

- Avoid fatigue and delayed-onset muscle soreness (24 to 48 hours postexercise) that can interfere with activities of daily living.

- Supervision by a trained professional is highly recommended, especially in the beginning when learning exercise technique and identifying safety issues.

- Program goals should address specific individual needs, such as locomotion in a wheelchair, transfers in and out of chairs or beds, and weight shifts, as in the case of paraplegia.

- Repetitive and exclusive use of upper body in performing activities of daily living can result in shoulder overuse injury and discomfort. Strengthening should focus on the upper back, chest, and shoulders, as well as stretching tight muscles around the shoulder joints.

- Circuit resistance training has been shown to be effective in those with paraplegia.

- Wheelchair users may need a strap or harness to stabilize the torso. Use brakes or sand bags against wheels to prevent tipping, particularly with overhead exercises.

Postpolio Syndrome See Neuromuscular Diseases

Stroke

- Strokes are closely associated with hypertension, and stroke victims may benefit from resistance training on both the affected and unaffected side (even the unaffected side is weaker than prior to a stroke as a result of both deconditioning and changes in motor pathways). Some believe resistance training interferes with coordination and timing in motor control, though this theory has not been supported by studies. Available studies suggest stroke victims can benefit substantially from resistance training by improving mobility, increasing functional capacity, reducing dependence on walking aids, and decreasing further disease risk. No clear resistance training guidelines exist at this time. Until they do, follow the General Guidelines for Those With Disabilities and Chronic Diseases (Table 2-3) adding the following precautions:

- Every effort should be made to avoid excessive, prolonged fatigue and delayed-onset muscle soreness (24 to 48 hours postexercise) that interferes with daily activities.

- For those with a low amount of functional muscle mass or severe weakness, performing resistance training without bands or weights may be sufficient initially (simply lifting an arm or leg against gravity and holding for 5 to 10 seconds may be an appropriate starting point).

- Assistance in lifting limbs and controlling movement against gravity may be necessary, at least in muscle groups that have had a severe loss of strength. Using adaptive gloves or velcro may help in securing a hand to a weight or bar.

- It may be impossible to exercise in a standing position. Modifications to assist with positioning, gripping, and coordination may need to be made. (Grips to be used with elastic bands can be purchased from online merchants such as Fitness Wholesale, www.fwonline.com.) Isometric exercise (a muscle squeeze with no movement in joints) of all responsive muscle may be most appropriate.

- Mental confusion or behavioral issues can be a factor affecting the ability to exercise.

- Additional medical complications common in older adults may also need to be accommodated, as the majority of strokes happen in the elderly. Assess for multiple medical conditions, and review the applicable guidelines for each condition listed in this section.

- Quality of movement must be given careful consideration. Individuals who have had a stroke sometimes tend to compensate for deficits by using *gross motor patterns* and using the wrong muscles in attempting to accomplish a movement (i.e., shrugging the shoulder during an arm lift). Consulting with a physical therapist or occupational therapist trained specifically in neurology is highly recommended.

- Blood pressure should be monitored closely, especially in the first month of exercise. Anyone who has had a stroke and continues to have unstable blood pressure should not exercise under any circumstances.

DOING IT

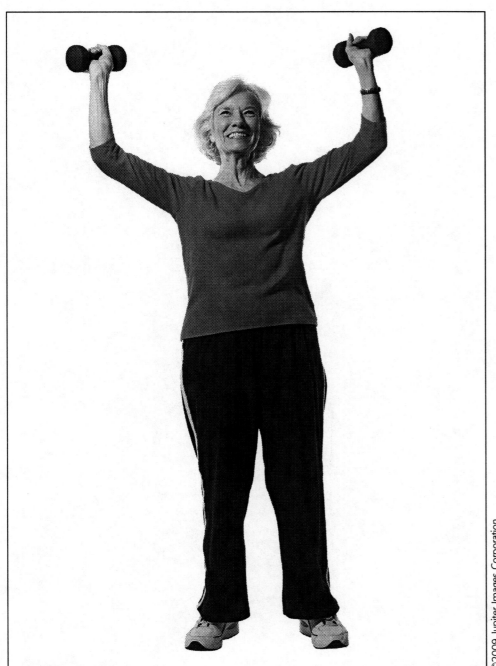

©2009 Jupiter Images Corporation

Part Two

3

Warming Up

First Things First: Posture and Breathing

Using Good Posture

Good posture is essential, not only when performing any exercise, but also when performing normal sitting and standing activities throughout the day.

Good posture will:

- Improve range of motion
- Increase breathing capacity
- Reduce the risk of falling
- Decrease the incidence of pain, especially in the lower back
- Reduce excessive load on joints and the spine

In general, posture should be:

- Upright, with the spine lifted (avoid slouching)
- Relaxed, not tense or rigid
- Focused on maintaining the natural curves of the spine (In other words, maintain a long spine, establishing the neutral low back curve.)

Good Seated Posture

Head/neck: Chin parallel to the floor, head in alignment with the spine, ears over the shoulders.

Shoulders: Relaxed and back.

Chest: Lifted and expanded.

Hips: Positioned at the back of the chair, not leaning against the back of the chair, which results in slumping and losing low back curve. If tired, place a rolled hand towel (about three inches in diameter) at low back to help maintain the natural curve.

Hands: Placed on thighs (while at rest).

Knees: Directly over ankles.

Feet: Flat on the floor, shoulder-distance apart, toes forward. If legs are not long enough for feet to reach the floor, slide hips toward the front of the chair or put a book or stool under the feet.

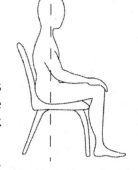

Figure 3-1. Good seated posture

Note: While this description details the "ideal" posture for sitting, be sure to shift sitting positions frequently (always maintaining neutral spine).

Good Standing Posture

Head/neck: Chin parallel to the floor, head in alignment with the spine, ears over the shoulders.

Shoulders: Relaxed and back.

Chest: Lifted and expanded.

Hips: Erect with a neutral low back curve. Check by placing hand at low back.

Hands: Relaxed by sides or resting lightly on the back of a chair for balance.

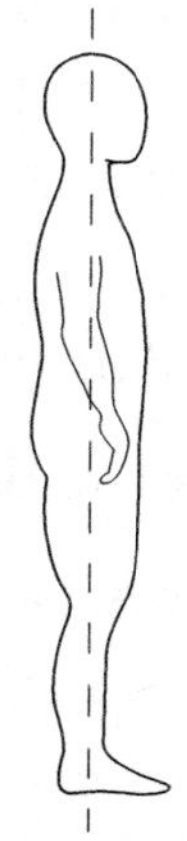

Figure 3-2. Good standing posture

Knees: Soft, not locked but not bent.

Feet: Shoulder-distance apart, toes forward.

Note: Shift standing position frequently.

Breathing

Contrary to popular belief, breathing does not always happen automatically. It is easy to hold your breath, especially while exercising and exerting. Use the following guidelines:

• Before beginning each exercise, be aware of your breathing.

• Breathe normally throughout exercises. Do not hold your breath.

• Those with pulmonary disease should practice pursed-lips breathing if it is helpful (see Appendix E).

Basic Warm-Up

Directions: Perform the following light, rhythmic physical activities to help safely prepare for more vigorous physical activity such as resistance training or aerobic exercise. These exercises can also be done for a quick, energizing "pick-me-up." This warm-up is especially valuable when combined with stretching exercises (see Chapter 5).

- *Duration:* 5-10 minutes (extend to 10-15 minutes if you are older, have a chronic disease/disability, or are significantly deconditioned). You can extend the time by adding the set of exercises from the "Basic Warm-Up for the Older Adult" section later in this chapter.

- *Pulmonary patients:* Accompany movements with pursed-lips breathing.

- Older adults or those unsteady on their feet: Exercises can be done seated. They may be combined with the set of exercises from the "Basic Warm-Up for the Older Adult" section later in this chapter.

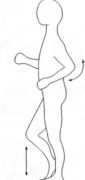

Walking in Place: 2-3 minutes

Instructions: Walk in place to increase inner core temperature and warm muscles. Start at a low intensity and increase gradually, using arms in a natural stride.

Figure 3-3

Wide Side-to-Side Knee Bend: 1 minute

Instructions: Place feet wider than shoulder width, with feet pointing out at a 45-degree angle. Bend one knee first and then the other, moving back and forth rhythmically. Do not bend the knee at more than a 90-degree angle, and less if you experience knee discomfort. Use support if necessary (e.g., the back of a chair) to help with balance. (If seated, just reach side to side with arms, pulling from the ribs.)

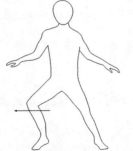

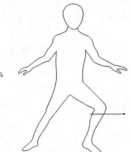

Figure 3-4   Figure 3-5

Rope Climb: 1 minute

Instructions: Place feet shoulder-width apart and reach toward the ceiling in a rope-climbing fashion, first with one arm and then the other. Lift the rib cage and shoulder

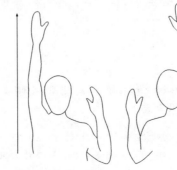

Figure 3-6

blade to feel a stretch throughout the torso. This exercise can be done sitting down if necessary.

Shoulder Rolls: 10 rolls, backward

Instructions: Lift shoulders toward ears and slowly roll in a full circle. Keep arms hanging at sides—avoid allowing elbows or hands to "take over." Roll backward for best posture benefit.

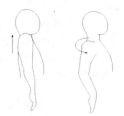

Figure 3-7

Arm Circles: 5 each arm, 5 together, backward

Instructions: Slowly rotate arm(s) backward using full pain-free range of motion. If necessary, make circles smaller or minimize how far back you circle to stay within pain tolerance. Rotate backward for best posture benefit.

Variation: Modify, if necessary, by placing hands on shoulders. Rotate elbows.

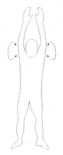 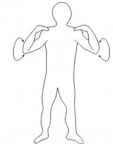

Figure 3-8

Figure 3-9. Variation

Basic Warm-Up for the Older Adult

Directions: Perform the following exercises with light intensity and rhythmic movements. You can choose to do some or all of the exercises. Warm up for a minimum of 5 to 10 minutes, preferably 10 to 15 minutes.

Note: The following exercises are not dangerous to underage adults—minors welcome.

Seated Walking in Place: 1-2 minutes

Instructions: Sit with good posture, maintaining the natural curves of the spine. Walk in place to increase inner core temperature and to warm the muscles. Start at a low intensity and increase gradually, using the arms in a natural stride.

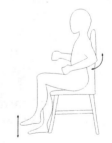

Figure 3-10

Seated Side Walking: Leg out and in, 5-10 each leg

Instructions: Sit with good posture, maintaining the natural curves of the spine. Move one leg out to the

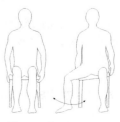

Figure 3-11

side, maintaining a 90-degree angle. Return to center. Alternate legs. This movement should come from the hip only, not the knee joint.

Seated Hip Circles: 5 in each direction, each leg

Instructions: Sit with good posture, maintaining the natural curves of the spine. Lift one foot a few inches off the floor. Draw circles with the knee, first in one direction, then the other. If necessary, rest the foot briefly before switching directions. Repeat with the other leg.

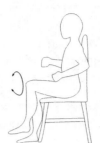

Figure 3-12

"Stir the Floor" With the Lower Leg: 5 in each direction, each leg

Instructions: Sit with good posture, maintaining the natural curves of the spine. Lift one foot a few inches off the floor. Rotate the leg from the knee, as though "stirring." Reverse directions. Repeat with the other leg.

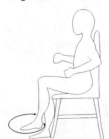

Figure 3-13

Ankle Rotations: 5-10 of each exercise, each foot

Instructions: Sit with good posture, maintaining the natural curves of the spine. Lift one foot a few inches off the floor. Draw circles with the foot, first in one direction, then the other. If necessary, rest the foot briefly before switching directions. Repeat with the other leg.

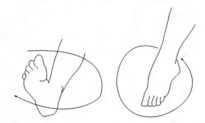

Figure 3-14

Variations:

- "Happy feet": Draw a smile (half-circle) with the foot in both directions.

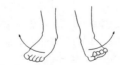

Figure 3-15

- Toe point/flex: Push toes forward, then pull back.

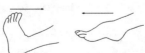

Figure 3-16

"Stir the Floor" With the Arm: 5 in each direction, both arms

Instructions: Sit with good posture, maintaining the natural curves of the spine. Lean slightly to one side, letting the arm hang down toward floor. Rotate the arm from the shoulder, "stirring the floor" with the arm. Reverse directions and switch arms.

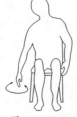

Figure 3-17

"Stir the Floor" With the Lower Arm: 5 in each direction, both arms

Instructions: Sit with good posture, maintaining the natural curves of the spine. Hold the upper arm to one side, letting the lower arm hang down toward the floor. Rotate the lower arm from the elbow, "stirring the floor" with the arm. Reverse directions and switch arms.

Note: If your shoulder hurts when holding your arm this way, hold your elbow at a lower position.

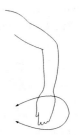
Figure 3-18

Wrist Rotations: 5 in each direction, both wrists

Instructions: Rotate the wrist in one direction, then reverse directions. Switch hands, or rotate simultaneously.

Figure 3-19

Elephant Ears Shoulder Exercise: 5-10 in each direction

Instructions: Clasp hands behind the head with the elbows straight out to the side. Keeping your hands in place, bring both elbows to the front so they are facing forward. Continue rhythmically, moving in full range of motion.

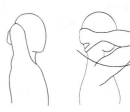
Figure 3-20

Seated Cat: 5-10 repetitions

Instructions: Sit with good posture, maintaining the natural curves of the spine. Press your lower back into the chair back (i.e., push your belly button into the lower part of the chair). Return to starting position. Move slowly and rhythmically.

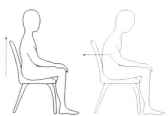
Figure 3-21

Seated Side-to-Side: 5-10 each side

Instructions: Sit with good posture, maintaining the natural curves of the spine. Hold on to the chair with one hand, while the opposite arm hangs straight at the side with palm facing in. Lower the hand toward the floor, returning to starting position. Repeat from the other side.

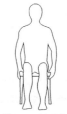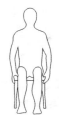
Figure 3-22

4

Strengthening

What's the Best Way to Strengthen Muscles?

Resistance training, as has been mentioned repeatedly throughout this book, is the most effective way to strengthen muscles. You may want to review the section on basic resistance training guidelines in Chapter 2 for more information. Various methods and types of equipment have been designed to effectively resistance train, including:

- Free weights (barbells and hand weights)
- Resistance machines (Nautilus®, Cybex®, Life Fitness®)
- Elastic resistance (bands, tubing)
- Simple calisthenics (effective especially when deconditioned or in the initial stages of resistance training)
- Household items (canned goods, sand-filled socks, bicycle inner tubes, jugs of water)

Using Elastic Resistance

Elastic resistance is the primary method of resistance training used in the exercises in this book. The author makes the assumption that not everyone has access—at least not all the time—to fitness facilities, nor a set of free weights at home. The bands provide an effective, yet easy and inexpensive, alternative ideal for a home program.

Elastic bands provide resistance by exerting muscles against a stretched elastic load. Many elastic resistance products are available that vary in shape, color, amount of resistance, and design. Regardless of the manufacturer of the elastic band, general resistance training principles apply (review Part One and read the section that follows). The exercises in this book are based on the use of a Thera-Band®, which is cut into four-foot lengths. Some exercises may need to be modified when using a different type of elastic band.

Advantages of Elastic Resistance

In general, older adults and novice resistance trainers have been encouraged by experts to use machines versus free weights when possible. The reason is that machines are sometimes regarded as safer to use and easier to learn, requiring less skill in controlling the exercise range of motion (ACSM Position Stand, 2002). While that assumption may be true, many older adults do not have access to machines. They need something they can use in their own homes, which is one of the many advantages to using elastic bands. Other advantages include the fact that they are:

- Easy to use, especially with practice
- Accommodating to many physical limitations
- Convenient in any location
- Light in weight, therefore portable and easy to take when you travel (even if just from room to room)
- Inexpensive
- Different colors (levels of resistance), providing easy opportunities for progression (See the following resistance equivalents.)
- Easy to modify the level of resistance (Slightly reducing slack or slightly increasing slack can accommodate a movement if necessary, though it is recommended to move to the next color when ready, rather than increasing the risk of breaking the band.)
- A convenient alternative to going to the gym'
- Able to be used while exercising in a standing position—which is good for bone density and muscle coordination

Using the Color-Coded System for the Right Level of Resistance

Most bands follow a color-coded system, providing a logical, easily individualized method of progression. Each color provides a different degree of resistance, making them accessible to a wide range of strength levels. In general, a 20 to 30 percent increase in force exists between each color level (more between silver and gold). The Thera-Band progression of resistance is shown in Table 4-1, starting with the thinnest bands with the least resistance, and progressing to the thickest bands with the most resistance.

A one-foot band elongated (stretched) to two feet would be a 100 percent elongation. If a four-foot band is doubled in length to eight feet, that would also be a 100 percent elongation.

It is unusual for one color of band to be appropriate for every exercise, as you have varying levels of strength in different muscle groups and varying

Color	Level of Resistance	Approximate Force in Pounds When Elongated (25 to 250 Percent)*
Tan	Extra light	Not available (less than yellow)
Yellow	Light resistance	1 to 6 pounds
Red	Medium	1 1/2 to 7 pounds
Green	Heavy	2 to 9 1/2 pounds
Blue	Extra heavy	3 to 13 pounds
Black	Special heavy	3 1/2 to 17 1/2 pounds
Silver	Super heavy	5 to 25 pounds
Gold	Max heavy	8 to 40 pounds

*Data from P. Page, A. Labbe, and R. Topp, *Journal of Orthopaedic & Sports Physical Therapy*, 30(1):A47-8, 2000.

Table 4-1. Thera-Band progression of resistance

degrees of muscle mass involved in each exercise. Color selection will also be impacted by potential disabilities or medical conditions. Review the general guidelines to find the appropriate color for each selected exercise. If you are initiating a program, it is wise to begin with a level of resistance that is less than what you think you can do. This method helps you to focus on developing your technique and also reduces the risk of injury.

Note: It is useful to practice exercises in front of a mirror. Correct form is extremely important, and mirrors provide ideal feedback.

Progressing With Elastic Resistance Exercise Bands

Keep in mind that to progress in muscular strength and endurance, the "overload principle" must be practiced, meaning you must safely but progressively overload the stress placed on the muscles. See the section on Guidelines for Progression later in this chapter for more information. With regard to the elastic bands specifically, once muscles have adapted to a certain color (level of resistance) and you plateau in progress, workload may be increased in one of the following ways:

• Progress to the elastic band with the next level of resistance.
• Use two elastic bands of the same color.
• Combine two colors of lower and higher resistance.

- Fold the band in half for exercises that accommodate this reduced length.
- For minor modifications in resistance, try adjusting grip position, alternating sides, or performing one side at a time.

Helpful Tips Using Elastic Resistance Bands

- Maintain the natural width of the band, keeping it open and flat, as much as possible to help prevent it from sliding or digging into skin.
- If the exercise requires a loop, make the loop about the size of your face. Tie it in a bow or half bow versus a knot to make it easier to untie. For added convenience, some people purchase extra bands to keep a permanent set of loops ready to use.
- Avoid wearing rings that can damage elastic bands. If you have long fingernails, try to keep them from cutting into the bands.
- Check bands for tears before using. Replace as necessary. If a band breaks, don't throw it away; you may be able to tie it in a permanent loop and continue using it.
- Protect your eyes while using bands.
- If you have a latex allergy, use latex-free bands.
- Store elastic bands out of direct sunlight, untied and flattened, folded, or hung. Periodically sprinkle bands with talcum powder.
- If you have arthritis or otherwise find the bands difficult to grip, handles can be purchased through providers such as Fitness Wholesale, www.fwonline.com Alternatively, you can try the free, often effective solution of tying a simple knot on each end of the band and cupping your fingers in the little pocket created next to the knot so that the knot is within your grip when you close your fist.

Reviewing Resistance Training Guidelines

Following are general exercise guidelines for exercise sessions and progression. Also refer to Tables 2-1, 2-2, and 2-4 for specific guidelines for special populations. Remember, these guidelines are not intended to replace specific instructions from your physician or specialist. Consult your physician before beginning your program if recommended when completing the PAR-Q in Appendix B.

Guidelines for Each Exercise Session: All Ages/All Fitness Levels

- Warm up before and cool down after each session, using the warming up exercises in Chapter 3 and the stretching exercises in Chapter 5.
- Maintain normal breathing—avoid holding breath.
- If a pulmonary condition is present, coordinate exercise movements with pursed-lips breathing. (See instructions in Appendix E.)

- Maintain the natural curves of the spine throughout each exercise (see the section on proper posture in Chapter 3).

- Use full, deliberate, controlled range of motion (one to two seconds in both directions).

- Resistance train two to three times per week on nonconsecutive days (two times per week is sometimes more appropriate).

- In general, follow the sequence of the exercises as presented in this book. The sequence follows the general principles of working large muscle groups before small, doing multiple-joint exercises before single-joint exercises, and alternating upper and lower body exercises.

- When adding target exercises to basic programs, follow the previous guideline describing optimal exercise sequence.

Guidelines for Progression

- Use light resistance for the first six to eight weeks (three to four weeks for younger individuals) to allow time for connective tissues to adapt to stress.

- Increase repetitions before increasing resistance (i.e., if you are on an 8 to 12 rep program, increase to 12 before adding resistance). When the last repetition is fairly light (RPE 11), add more resistance (i.e., the next level colored band), and drop back to 8 to 10 repetitions.

- If 8 to 10 repetitions cannot be performed in good form, the resistance is too heavy.

- When adding resistance or if adding an additional set, reduce repetitions to 10, and gradually progress to 15 based on exertion.

- In general, strive for a perceived exertion of somewhat hard (RPE 12 to 13). If you have been consistent, have established a good foundation (at least 6 to 12 weeks), and are experiencing no symptoms, you may increase your effort level up to hard (RPE 15). Maximal effort (RPE 19 to 20) on the last repetition is appropriate for *healthy* adults under the age of 50 to 60 who have followed a gradual, safe, consistent progression. See RPE scale in Appendix D.

- Increases should range from 2 to 10 percent at a time—greater increases for exercises using large muscle groups and multiple joints (i.e., squats, chest presses), and smaller increases for exercises using small muscle groups and single joints (i.e., leg extensions, bicep curls).

- Variation becomes important in long-term resistance training, so vary the amount of resistance, number of repetitions, speed of repetitions, rest periods, number of sets, total volume, and selection of exercises.

Precautions

- Always maintain a neutral lower-back curve to protect the back (see section on posture in Chapter 3).

- Do not push through pain. In the event of pain, perform the exercise with no resistance, or, if using an elastic band, give yourself more slack. Seek assistance if in doubt.

- *Stop* resistance training and notify someone immediately if you have any of the following symptoms: dizziness, abnormal heart rhythm, unusual shortness of breath, or chest pain. Seek assistance from a health professional.

- Use proper form when doing all exercises. Practice in front of a mirror to check yourself. Ideally, an appropriately trained individual can assist you.

Resistance Training Programs: Which Is Yours?

The following lists of exercises summarize the programs in this chapter, described in detail and accompanied by illustrations. The basic resistance programs are designed to be complete programs, including all the major muscle groups in the body. The target programs are intended for areas of concern or added interest, and can be folded into a basic group (making substitutions so that each program consists of only 12 exercises). Or you may do a basic program on one day, and a selection of target exercises on alternate days. See which method works best for you. Be sure to list your program on the Resistance Training Log shown in Appendix N.

Basic: Just Starting
- Abdominal squeeze
- Thigh squeeze
- Straight-leg raise
- Seated row
- Chest press
- Bicep curl
- Tricep extension
- Stand-up

Basic: Maintenance #1
- Squat
- Abdominal curl
- Back extension
- Leg extension
- Hamstring curl
- Bent-over row
- Chest press
- Lat pull-down
- Upright row
- Shoulder press

Basic: Maintenance #2
- Leg press
- Seated abdominal or overhead crunch
- Rotary torso
- Pull-over
- Reverse fly
- Chest fly
- Tricep press
- Bicep curl
- Frontal raise

Basic: In the Chair
- Abdominal squeeze
- Thigh squeeze
- Straight-leg raise #1
- Straight-leg raise #2
- Leg press
- Seated chest press
- Seated upright row
- Seated bent-over row
- Shoulder press
- Standup

Basic: In Bed
- Straight-leg raise
- Abdominal squeeze
- Leg extension
- Leg curl
- Chest press
- Upright row
- Bicep curl
- Tricep extension
- Frontal raise
- Ankle rotation
- Wrist rotation

Target: Abdominal
- Abdominal squeeze
- Abdominal curl
- Abdominal leg extension
- Seated abdominal
- Overhead abdominal crunch
- Rotary torso
- Side bend
- Side bridge

Target: For the Back
- Slow lunge
- Abdominal curl
- Single-leg extension hold
- Side bridge

Target: Hips, Knees, and Ankles
- Hip extension
- Hip abduction
- Hip adduction
- Stepping
- Thigh squeeze
- Straight-leg raise #1
- Straight-leg raise #2
- Terminal extension
- Leg extension
- Hamstring curl
- Calf raise
- Toe pull
- Ankle rotation
- Happy feet
- Toe point/flex

Target: Peripheral Arterial Disease
- Stepping
- Hip extension
- Hip abduction
- Hip adduction
- Squat
- Calf raise

Target: Shoulder
- Bent-over row
- Shoulder diagonal sweep (high to low)
- Shoulder cross diagonal sweep (high to low)
- Shoulder cross diagonal sweep (low to high)
- Rotary cuff #1
- Rotary cuff #2
- Rotary cuff #3

Target: Chest/Breast Surgery
- Abdominal strengthener
- Hand lean
- Lateral raise
- Frontal raise
- Bicep curl
- Shoulder extension
- Tricep press
- Hands and knees
- Serratus reach
- Lower back bridge

Target: Osteoporosis
- Stepping
- Hip extension
- Hip abduction/adduction
- Back extension
- Squat
- Slow lunge
- Seated row
- Lat pull-down
- Pull-over
- Bicep curl
- Wrist curl
- Reverse wrist curl
- Wrist rotation

Basic Resistance Training Program:
Just Starting

Frequency: 2-3 times per week on nonconsecutive days (unless otherwise advised)

Intensity: Low to moderate (RPE 11-13) initially, gradually progressing to moderate to hard (RPE 13-15) as tolerated (unless otherwise advised)

Repetitions: 10-15 (unless otherwise advised)

Sets: 1 set minimum, increasing gradually to 2-3 if tolerated (unless otherwise advised)

Rest Periods: 1-2 minutes between sets (unless otherwise advised) (see Chapter 2)

Progression: Every 2-4 weeks, or longer based on tolerance. As this program is intended for beginners, progress at no more than 2-5 percent at a time. See the Guidelines for Progression discussed previously in this chapter for more information.

This program is especially designed for:

- People just starting resistance training (to be followed for a three-month period)
- Deconditioned adults
- Older adults
- People with arthritis, fibromyalgia, or chronic fatigue syndrome
- People with any condition that calls for a slow, easy initial program

Note: Review the specific guidelines for each condition in Chapter 2.

If arthritis or fibromyalgia is present:

- Reduce the number of repetitions to start (this precaution should also be taken if you are older and very deconditioned).
- Begin with very light resistance (RPE 8-11).
- Resistance train only two times per week on nonconsecutive days.
- Use light resistance for the first six to eight weeks to allow time for connective tissues to adapt to stress and to evaluate tolerance to resistance training.
- Increase repetitions before increasing resistance.
- Progress very slowly—no more than 2 to 5 percent at a time or 10 percent per week.
- If all repetitions cannot be performed in good form, the resistance is too heavy and should be lowered.
- Be conservative when involving painful joints.
- Do not exacerbate pain. Do not use added resistance during flare-ups.

If chronic fatigue syndrome or severe deconditioning is present:

- Begin with very light resistance (RPE 8-11).
- Try doing aerobic exercise on alternate days rather than on the same day of resistance training.
- Use no resistance to start, using only your own body weight. Consider not adding any resistance (i.e., bands) until you can do three sets of 15 repetitions, performed throughout the day if necessary.

Abdominal Squeeze

Purpose: Improves strength of abdominal muscles to help stabilize the spine

Instructions: Sit in a chair and maintain good posture. Place hands on thighs near the knees. Push down firmly on the thighs while tightening the abdominal muscles. Maintain a neutral lower-back curve. Hold for three to five seconds. Repeat.

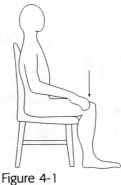

Figure 4-1

Note: This exercise can also be done while lying on the floor or bed with the knees bent (Figure 4-2).

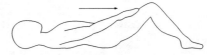

Figure 4-2. Lying down

Variation: Repeat instructions for Abdominal Squeeze, but place both hands on one thigh near the knee, while turning the opposite shoulder toward hands. Hold for three to five seconds. Repeat.

Note: This variation can also be done while lying on the floor or bed with the knees bent.

Caution: Avoid overtwisting.

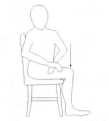

Figure 4-3. Variation

Thigh Squeeze

Purpose: Improves strength of quadricep muscles and helps stabilize the knee

Instructions: Sit with hips toward the front of a chair. Extend one leg straight out, toes pointing up, heel resting on the floor. Tighten thigh muscle of the extended leg. Hold for three to five seconds. Repeat.

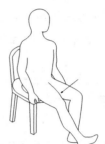

Figure 4-4

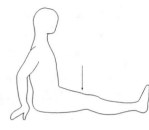

Figure 4-5. Seated on the floor or in bed

Note: This exercise can also be done sitting on the floor or in a bed.

Straight-Leg Raise

Purpose: Improves strength of quadricep muscles and helps stabilize the knee

Instructions: Sit with hips toward the front of a chair. Extend one leg straight out, toes pointing up, heel resting on the floor. Keeping the knee straight, raise the extended

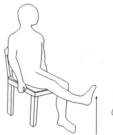

Figure 4-6

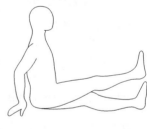

Figure 4-7. Seated on the floor or in bed

leg so it is parallel to the floor. Hold for three to five seconds. Return to the start position and repeat. Note: This exercise can also be done sitting on the floor or in a bed.

Seated Row

Purpose: Strengthens biceps and upper back

Instructions: Sit in a chair with one leg extended. Loop a band across the sole of the extended foot. Grasp the band in each hand about 12 inches from the foot on each side, taking up excess slack.

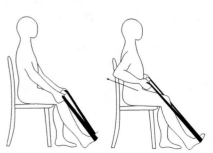

Figure 4-8

Maintain a neutral lower-back curve. Pull both elbows straight back to full flexion. Return to the start position and repeat.

Note: This exercise can also be done sitting on the floor or in a bed.

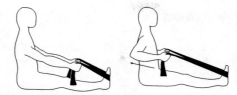

Figure 4-9. Seated on the floor or in bed

Chest Press

Purpose: Strengthens triceps, pectorals (chest), and deltoids (shoulders)

Instructions: Position a band across the shoulder blades. Keep the band open and flat. With the band taut, grasp the band at each underarm. Extend the arms fully, keeping parallel to each other and to the floor. Return to the start position and repeat.

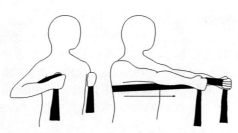

Figure 4-10. Seated on the floor or in bed

Bicep Curl

Purpose: Strengthens biceps

Instructions: Hold one end of a band in each hand. Step on the middle of the band. Hang arms straight at sides, thumb-side of hand facing forward. "Glue" elbows to ribs. Fully flex one arm at a time or both arms together. Return to the start position and repeat.

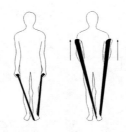

Figure 4-11

Tricep Extension

Purpose: Strengthens triceps

Instructions: Hold one end of an elastic band and tuck it just under the chin. Grasp the band about 6 to 12 inches below that point with the other hand. "Glue" both elbows to ribs. Keeping one hand tucked under the chin and elbows against ribs, fully straighten the arm of the other hand. Return to the start position and repeat.

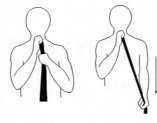

Figure 4-12

Stand-up

Purpose: Strengthens quadriceps, improves the ability to rise from a seated position

Instructions: Sit in a chair with feet shoulder-width apart. With minimal use of hands and minimal leaning forward, slowly stand to full extension. Return slowly to start position and repeat.

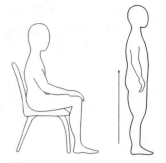

Figure 4-13

Note: If knee pain, thigh weakness, or instability is experienced, try sitting on something (such as a phone book) that elevates you two to four inches. If you need further assistance to stand, place a chair or walker in front of you. Minimize reliance on this device when possible, but use if necessary.

Variation: When stand-ups are no longer challenging, use a band for more resistance. Stand on a band with one or both feet, pick up slack until the band is taut, and stand as shown in Figure 4-14.

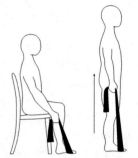

Figure 4-14. Variation

Basic Resistance Training Program: Maintenance #1

Frequency: 2-3 times per week on nonconsecutive days (unless otherwise advised)

Intensity: Moderate (RPE 12-13) initially, increasing to moderate to high (RPE 13-15) as tolerated (unless otherwise advised)

Repetitions: 8-12 if healthy and less than 50-60 years; otherwise 10-15

Sets: 1 set initially, increasing gradually to 2 or 3 as tolerated (unless otherwise advised)

Rest periods: 2-3 minutes between exercises using heavier loads, large muscle groups, and multiple joints; 1-2 minutes for "assistance" exercises using smaller muscle groups and single joints (see Chapter 2)

Progression: Every 1-3 weeks for younger individuals, every 2-4 weeks for older or more deconditioned individuals (or longer based on tolerance). Progression should not be more than 2-10 percent increase at a time (with the higher range for exercises using larger muscle groups and multiple joints, and the lower range for exercises using small muscle groups and single joints). The greatest long-term returns occur when effort is gradually increased to maximal (RPE 19-20), if safely tolerated. Variation becomes important in long-term resistance training. See the Guidelines for Progression discussed previously in this chapter.

This program is especially designed for:

- Healthy individuals
- People who have been doing the basic "Just Starting" program and are ready for more
- People who have been doing "Maintenance #2" and want variety or are "periodizing" their program (see Chapter 2)
- People able to perform the following exercises successfully

Note: Please review the specific guidelines in Chapter 2, and check to see if you have any condition that may result in necessary modifications.

For variation, rotate every four to eight weeks between this program and Maintenance #2 to help avoid boredom and the plateau in progression that is often seen with programs that do not incorporate variation.

Squat

Purpose: Strengthens primarily the quadriceps and gluteals

Instructions: Step on a band with one foot or two (using both feet adds more resistance). Pick up the slack so the band is taut. Stand with good posture—feet shoulder-width apart or slightly wider, toes turned out to a 45-degree angle, arms straight at the sides. Bend both knees to about a 45-degree angle (no more than a 90-degree angle), or within knee stability range. Weight will be primarily over the heels of the feet. Do not lean your torso forward—remain upright. Return to the start position and repeat.

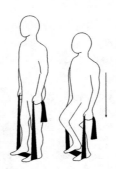

Figure 4-15

Abdominal Curl

Purpose: Strengthens abdominal muscles

Instructions: Lay on your back on a firm surface with knees bent. Place your hands under your lower back to stabilize the pelvis and maintain a neutral spine. Raise your head and shoulders off the ground. Return to the start position and repeat. For more resistance, you may hold a hand weight or other easily managed load against your chest. Be sure to maintain a neutral lower-back curve as your hands will be holding weight.

Figure 4-16

Variations:

- Keep one leg straight to help maintain a neutral lower-back curve (Figure 4-17).

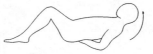

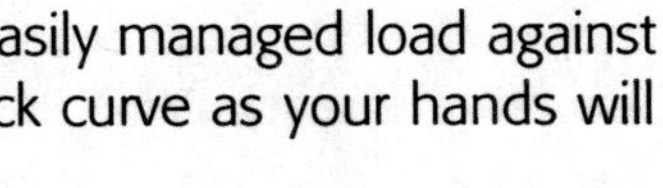

Figure 4-17. Variation

• To promote abdominal strength and endurance, start in the standard abdominal curl position, and curl to the right, then to the left. (Not pictured. See Figure 4-16 for reference.)

Back Extension

Purpose: Strengthens back muscles

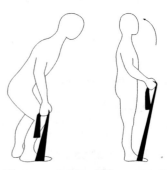

Instructions: Step on a band with one foot or two (using both feet adds more resistance). Grasp each end of the band in each hand. Pick up the slack so the band is taut. Lean forward to approximately a 45-degree angle, bending from the hips and maintaining a neutral lower-back curve. Keeping your elbows straight, carefully erect your torso to an upright position. Return to the start position and repeat.

Figure 4-18.   Figure 4-19.
Standing   Seated

Note: It is *very* important not to round the back when doing this exercise. Do *not* include this exercise if you have an acute back injury or back pain. This exercise can be performed sitting or standing.

Leg Extension

Purpose: Strengthens quadriceps

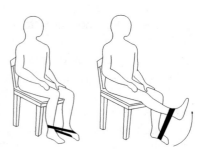

Instructions: Tie the band in a loop. Step on the band with one foot, anchoring the band on the floor during the exercise. Loop the band around the other ankle (i.e., the leg that will exercise first). Sit with both legs at a 90-degree angle. Tuck both hands under the thigh of the leg you will use first. Fully straighten the leg, pausing at full extension. Return to the start position and repeat.

Figure 4-20

Hamstring Curl

Purpose: Strengthens hamstrings

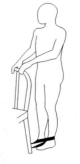

Instructions: Stand behind a chair or some type of support. Tie the band in a loop. Stand on loop with one leg, and position the band around the other ankle. Bending the knee of that leg, pull the heel toward your hip to a 90-degree angle. Keep your knee pointing toward the floor. Avoid allowing the knee to "pull forward." Return to the start position and repeat.

Figure 4-21

Bent-Over Row

Purpose: Strengthens biceps and upper back muscles, stabilizes shoulder joint

Instructions: Grasp each end of a band in each hand. Step on the middle of the band. Bend torso forward and rest your hand (on the same side

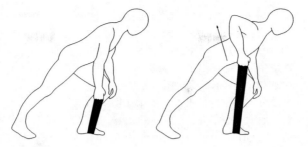

Figure 4-22

as your forward leg) on your knee for support (or use the back of a chair, counter, or table for support). Straighten the other arm toward the floor. Take excess slack out of the band as needed. Pull your elbow (not your hand) toward the ceiling in full flexion. Return to the start position and repeat.

Note: Be sure the upper body is supported to protect your back. Avoid forward flexion if you have osteoporosis.

Chest Press

Purpose: Strengthens triceps, pectorals, and deltoids

Instructions: Position a band across your shoulder blades. Try to keep the band open and flat. Maintain a neutral lower-back curve. Grasp the band at each underarm—*not* at the

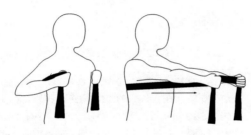

Figure 4-23

ends of the band (allow plenty of slack). Extend your arms fully, keeping them parallel to each other and to the floor. Return to the start position and repeat.

Lat Pull-down

Purpose: Strengthens primarily the latissimus dorsi (mid-back) and biceps

Instructions: Anchor the middle of a band to a secure overhead hook or bar (a bicycle hook or chin-up bar works well), or tie a knot in the center of a band and shut the knot on the other side of the top of a

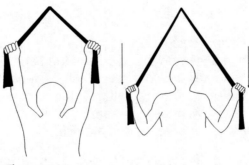

Figure 4-24

door. Grasp each end of the band in each hand, picking up slack so the arms are fully extended overhead (you may want to sit in a chair to accomplish this movement). Pull the elbows toward the ribs, fully flexing the arms. Return to the start position and repeat.

Modified Lat Pull-down (if overhead anchor is not available): Grasp the band overhead with arms fully extended and hands about 18 inches apart. Pulling your elbows to your ribs, flex the elbows as you pull your hands apart, lowering the band in front of your face. Return to the start position and repeat.

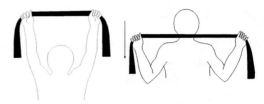

Figure 4-25. Modified: no overhead anchor

Variation: Lower your arms out to your sides without bending your elbows, so that your arms are straight and parallel to the floor and the band is in front of your body. Return to the start position and repeat.

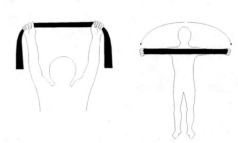

Figure 4-26. Variation: keeping elbows straight

Upright Row

Purpose: Strengthens deltoids and biceps

Instructions: Grasp each end of a band in each hand. Step on the middle of the band. Stand with arms straight, hands together, and palms facing your body. Lift both hands to your chin, keeping your hands together, and leading with the elbows. Return to the start position and repeat.

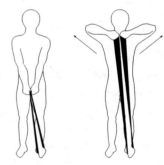

Figure 4-27

Shoulder Press

Purpose: Strengthens deltoids and triceps

Instructions: Grasp each end of a band in each hand. Step on the middle of the band. Bring one hand to shoulder level. Fully extend that arm toward the ceiling. Return to the start position and repeat with the other arm. If well tolerated, both arms can be extended at once.

Note: If resistance is too high to allow full extension and you do not have a band with less resistance, increase the slack on the side you are using.

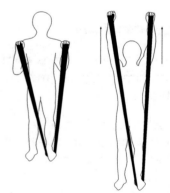

Figure 4-28

Basic Resistance Training Program:
Maintenance #2

Frequency: 2-3 times per week on nonconsecutive days (unless otherwise advised)

Intensity: Moderate (RPE 12-13) initially, increasing to moderate to high (RPE 13-15) as tolerated (unless otherwise advised). Greatest returns long-term occur when effort is gradually increased to maximal (RPE 19-20), if safely tolerated

Repetitions: 8-12 if healthy and less than 50-60 years; otherwise 10-15

Sets: 1 set initially, increasing gradually to 2 or 3 as tolerated (unless otherwise advised)

Rests: 2-3 minutes between exercises using heavier loads and using large muscle groups and multiple joints; 1-2 minutes for "assistance" exercises using smaller muscle groups and single joints (see Chapter 2)

Progression: Every 1-3 weeks for younger individuals, every 2-4 weeks for older or more deconditioned individuals (or longer based on tolerance); no more than a 2-10 percent increase at a time (the higher end of that range for exercises using larger muscle groups and multiple joints; the lower end of that range for exercises using small muscle groups and single joints). Variation becomes important in long-term resistance training. See the Guidelines for Progression discussed previously in this chapter.

This program is especially designed for:

- Healthy individuals
- People who have been doing the basic "Just Starting" program and are ready for more
- People who have been doing "Maintenance #1" and want variety or are "periodizing" their program (see Chapter 2)
- People able to perform the exercises listed below successfully

Note: Please review specific guidelines in Chapter 2, and check to see if you have any specific condition discussed that may describe modifications for you.

For variation, rotate every four to eight weeks between this program and "Maintenance #1" to help to avoid boredom and the plateau in progression that is often seen with programs that do not incorporate variation.

Leg Press

Purpose: Strengthens primarily the quadriceps and gluteals

Instructions: Sit with one thigh pulled toward the chest. Position a band across the ball of your foot. Grasp the band in each hand about 12 inches from your ankle on each side, picking up slack so that the band is taut. Keeping the arms stationary, extend your leg so it is completely parallel to floor. Return to the start position and repeat.

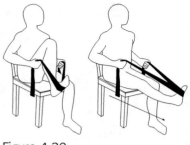

Figure 4-29

Note: Greater resistance can often be used on this exercise. Try doubling the band or combining two bands together.

Seated Abdominal or Overhead Abdominal Crunch

❏ Seated Abdominals

Purpose: Strengthens abdominals

Instructions:

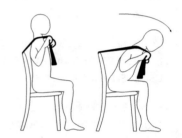

Figure 4-31. Preferred method: band over the shoulders (anchor required)

- Preferred method: Choose a chair that has a handle at the top of the chair back. Sit in the chair with good posture. Thread the band through the handle and bring the band over each shoulder. The band should be taut. Bending from your hips, lean torso over thighs. Return to the start position and repeat.

- Alternative method: If the chair has no handle, position the band across the chair back and tuck the band under each underarm. The band should be taut. Bending from your hips, lean torso over thighs. Return to the start position and repeat.

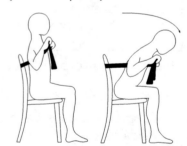

Figure 4-32. Alternative method: band under arms (band across back of chair)

Note: Greater resistance can often be used on this exercise. Try doubling the band or combining two bands together.

Note: Use caution with forward flexion if you have osteoporosis. Maintain neutral spine, keeping chest lifted.

❏ Overhead Abdominal Crunches

Purpose: Strengthens abdominals and the internal and external obliques

Instructions: Anchor the middle of a band to a secure overhead hook or bar such as a bicycle hook or a chin-up bar. You could also tie a knot in the center of a band and shut the knot on the other side of the top of a door. Sit in a chair with good posture, positioned directly below the anchor. Grasp each end of the band in each hand and bring your hands to your shoulders, palms facing out. Keeping your hands at your shoulders, "shorten" your torso by tightening your abdominal muscles and bringing your chest closer to your thighs.

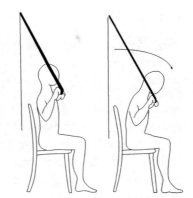

Figure 4-33

Variation: Rotate toward your right thigh, and then rotate toward your left thigh.

Rotary Torso

Purpose: Strengthens abdominals and internal and external obliques

Instructions: Sit in a chair. Anchor a band around one arm of the chair, or, if your chair doesn't have an arm, around the outermost side bar of the chair back. Sit with good posture. Rotate torso toward the band, being careful not to overtwist. Grasp the band with both hands about six inches from the chair frame. Using your abdominal muscles—not your hands—rotate torso to a forward-facing position. Return to the start position and repeat.

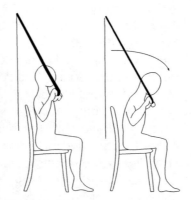

Figure 4-34

Pull-Over

Purpose: Strengthens the latissimus dorsi, triceps, and chest muscles

Instructions: Anchor the middle of a band to a secure overhead hook or bar such as a bicycle hook or a chin-up bar. You could also tie a knot in the center of a band and shut the knot on the other side of the top of a door. Stand below the anchor. Grasp each end of the band in each hand, so that your arms are nearly fully extended overhead, elbows slightly flexed and palms facing each other. Lower your arms to your sides, ending with your elbows at your ribs and bent to 90-degree angle. Return to the start position and repeat.

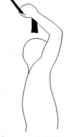

Figure 4-35

Reverse Fly

Purpose: Strengthens the latissimus dorsi, trapezius (upper back), and back of deltoids

Instructions: Grasp a band in each hand about 12 inches apart. Stand with your arms straight out in front of you, parallel to the floor and to each other. Keeping elbows straight, bring both arms out to the side and parallel to floor. Return to the start position and repeat.

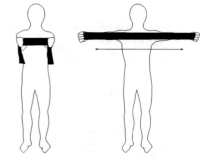

Figure 4-36

Chest Fly

Purpose: Strengthens pectorals and front of deltoids

Instructions: Anchor a band to a secure hook, bar, or railing at shoulder height. You could also tie a knot at one end of the band and shut the knot on the other side of a door at shoulder height. Stand with feet shoulder-width apart (or a bit more) beside the anchor. Grasp the band with the hand that is nearest to the anchor. Stand with that arm slightly flexed and parallel to the floor, palm facing out. Bring arm toward

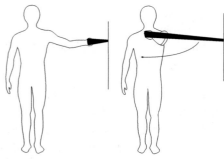

Figure 4-37

the midline of your body, keeping it parallel to the floor and the elbow only slightly flexed. Return to the start position and repeat.

Tricep Press: Variation #1 or #2

Purpose: Strengthens triceps

Instructions:

Variation #1: Hold one end of a band against your chin. Grasp the band with the other hand 6 to 12 inches from the first hand and tuck that elbow against your ribs. Keeping the first hand against your chin and your elbow against your ribs, extend your arm completely until your hand is against the side of your body. Return to the start position and repeat.

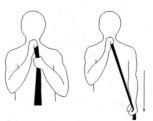

Figure 4-38

Variation #2: Anchor the middle of a band to a secure overhead hook or bar. Or, tie a knot in the center of the band and shut the knot on the other side of the door. Stand below the anchor. Grasp each end of the band in each hand. Keeping both elbows against the ribs, fully extend your arms. Return to the start position and repeat.

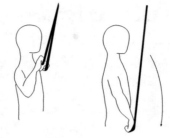

Figure 4-39. Variation #2

Bicep Curl

Purpose: Strengthens biceps

Instructions: Step on the middle of a band with one foot. Grasp each end of the band in each hand. Stand with your arms straight at your sides, palms facing the body. Keeping your elbows "glued" to your ribs, fully flex both arms. Return to the start position and repeat.

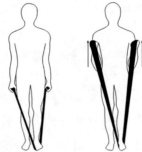

Figure 4-40

Frontal/Lateral Raise

Purpose: Strengthens deltoids

Instructions:

Part 1 (Frontal Raise): Step on the middle of a band with one foot. Grasp each end of the band in each hand. Stand with your arms straight at your sides, backs of hands facing forward. Raise both arms in front of your body until they are parallel to the floor, keeping your elbows straight. Return to the start position.

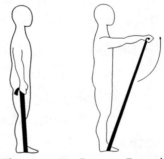

Figure 4-41. Part 1: Frontal raise

Part 2 (Lateral Raise): Face palms toward the body. Raise both arms out to your sides until parallel to the floor, with palms facing the floor. Return to the start position and repeat Part 1.

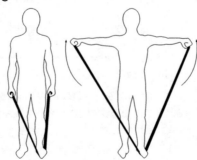

Figure 4-42. Part 2: Lateral raise

Basic Resistance Training Program: In the Chair

Frequency: 2-3 times per week on nonconsecutive days (unless otherwise advised).

Intensity: Low to moderate initially (RPE 11-13), gradually progressing to moderate to hard (RPE 13-15) as tolerated (unless otherwise advised).

Repetitions: 10-15 (unless otherwise advised).

Sets: 1 set initially; increasing gradually to 2-3 if tolerated (unless otherwise advised).

Rest Periods: 1-2 minutes between sets, unless otherwise advised (Chapter 2).

Progression: Every 2-4 weeks, or longer based on tolerance; no more than 2-5 percent at a time (Chapter 2).

Special: For best results, combine with "Basic Stretching Program: In the Chair" (Chapter 5).

This program is especially designed for:

- Difficulty standing or unable to stand
- Balance problems
- Older adults
- Arthritis, fibromyalgia, chronic fatigue syndrome
- Stroke
- Physical disabilities (persons in a wheelchair, etc)
- Other conditions that make someone feel more comfortable in a chair

    Please review specific guidelines for each condition in Part One.

Note: While it may be necessary and/or a good idea from a safety standpoint to exercise while seated, try standing when possible. Standing allows the accessory muscles (those muscles trying to hold you up as you move through the exercises) to work, improving balance and coordination, and it is more effective. Standing while performing resistance-training exercises also has more impact on bone mineral density. However, if you are at risk of falling, unduly fatigued, and/or significantly short of breath, please remain seated while exercising.

Abdominal Squeeze

Purpose: Improves strength of abdominal muscles to help stabilize spine.

Instructions: Sit in a chair. Place hands on thighs near knees. Push down firmly on thighs while tightening abdominal muscles. Maintain neutral low back curve. Hold for three to five seconds. Repeat.

Note: This exercise can also be done lying on the floor or bed with knees bent.

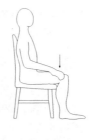

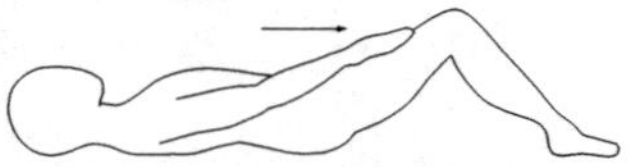

Figure 4-43

Variation: Repeat previous directions, but place both hands on one thigh near knee, while turning opposite shoulder toward hands. Hold for three to five seconds. Repeat.

Figure 4-44. Lying down

Note: This exercise can also be done lying on the floor or bed with knees bent.

Caution: Avoid overtwisting.

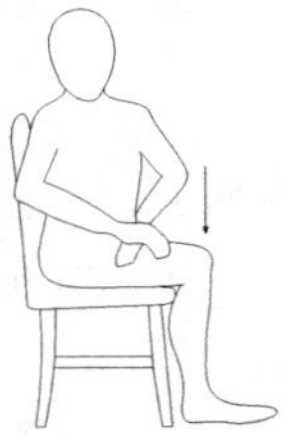

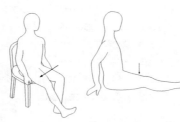

Figure 4-45. Variation

Quadriceps (Front of Thigh) Series

The following four exercises are to strengthen the front of the thigh. They can be done in sequence, switching legs each time, or interspersed with arm exercises if muscle fatigue is not well tolerated. These exercises are good for stabilizing the knee joint. The first three are especially well-tolerated, as they do not require flexing the knee joint.

❑ Thigh Squeeze

Instructions: Sit with hips toward front of chair. Extend one leg straight in front of you, with toes pointing up and heel resting on the floor. Tighten thigh muscle of the extended leg. Hold for three to five seconds. Repeat.

Note: This exercise can also be done sitting on the floor or in bed.

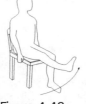

Figure 4-46

Figure 4-47. Seated on the floor

❑ Straight Leg Raise #1 (holding)

Instructions: Sit with hips toward front of chair. Extend one leg straight in front of you, with your toes pointing up and your heel resting on the floor. Keeping your knee straight, raise extended leg to parallel to the floor. Hold for three to five seconds. Return to the start position and repeat.

Figure 4-48

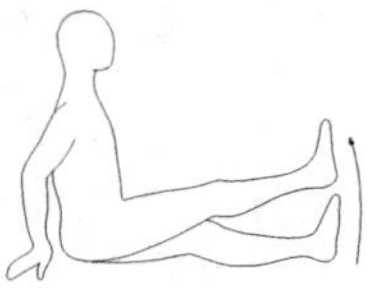

Figure 4-49. Seated on the floor

Note: This exercise can also be done sitting on the floor or in bed.

❑Straight Leg Raise #2

Instructions: Sit with your hips toward the front of a chair. Extend one leg straight in front of you, with your toes pointing up and your heel resting on the floor. Keeping your knee straight,

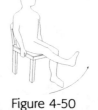
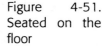

Figure 4-50

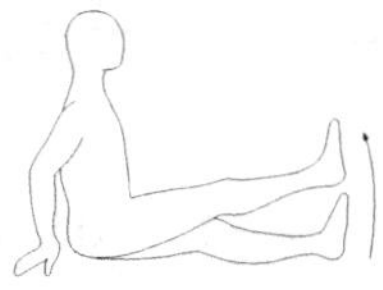

Figure 4-51. Seated on the floor

perform as in previous exercise, raising extended leg to parallel to floor, but don't hold. Return to the start position and repeat.

Note: This exercise can also be done sitting on the floor or in bed.

❑Leg Press

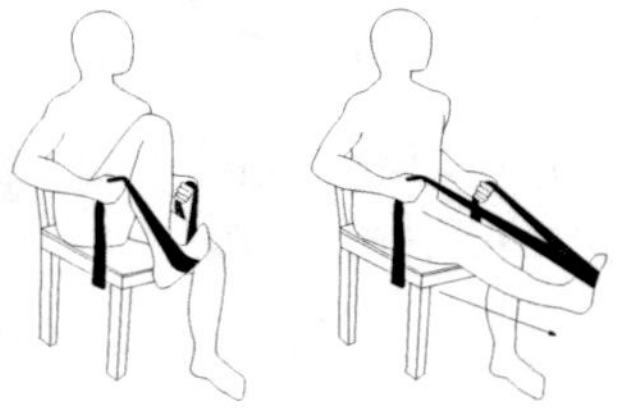

Instructions: Sit in chair. Pull one thigh toward your chest. Fully extend the leg until it is parallel to the floor. Return to the start position and repeat.

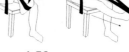

Figure 4-52

Note: This exercise can add band when appropriate. See Maintenance #2 earlier in this chapter for specific instructions.

Seated Chest Press

Purpose: Strengthens triceps (back of upper arm), pectorals (chest), and deltoids (shoulders).

Instructions: Sit in a chair with your hips toward front of chair and shoulders supported against chair back. Position band across shoulder blades. Maintain neutral lower-back curve. With band taut, grasp at each underarm. Extend your arms fully, keeping parallel to each other and to the floor. Return to the start position and repeat.

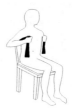
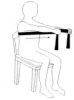

Figure 4-53

Seated Upright Rows

Purpose: Strengthens deltoids (top of shoulders) and biceps (front of upper arm).

Instructions: Grasp end of the band in each hand. Step on middle of the band. Sit with knees apart and arms straight between the knees, hands together, and palms facing your body. Lift both hands to chin level, leading with the elbows and fully flexing both arms. Return to the start position and repeat.

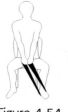
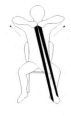

Figure 4-54

Seated Bent-Over Row

Purpose: Strengthens biceps (front of upper arm) and upper-back muscles, stabilizes shoulder joint.

Instructions: Sit in a chair. Grasp end of the band in each hand. Step on middle of the band. Bend torso forward, and rest one elbow on your knee for support. Straighten other arm with hand toward floor between

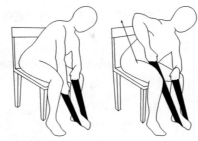

Figure 4-55

knees. Take excess slack out of the band. Pull your elbow (not hand) toward the ceiling in full flexion. Return to the start position and repeat. Use caution with forward flexion if you have osteoporosis.

Shoulder Press

Purpose: Strengthens deltoids (top of shoulders) and triceps (back of upper arm).

Instructions: Grasp end of the band in each hand. Step on middle of the band. Bring one hand to shoulder level. Fully extend your arm toward ceiling. Return to the start position and repeat. If well tolerated, you can use both arms at once.

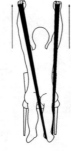
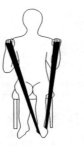

Figure 4-56

Stand-Ups

Purpose: Strengthens quadriceps (front of thigh), and improves ability to get out of chair.

Instructions: Sit in a chair with your feet shoulder-width apart. With minimal use of hands and minimal leaning forward, slowly stand to full extension. Return slowly to the start position and repeat.

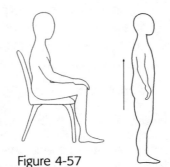

Figure 4-57

If you have knee pain or thigh weakness, or if instability is experienced, try sitting on something that elevates you 2 to 4 inches, such as a phone book. If you need further assistance to stand, place chair or walker in front of you. Minimize reliance on assistance when possible, but use if necessary.

Variation: When stand-ups are no longer challenging, use a band for more resistance: stand on the band with one or both feet, pick up slack until the band is taut, and stand as shown in Figure 4-58.

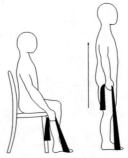

Figure 4-58. Variation

Basic Resistance Training Program: In Bed

Frequency: As tolerated—consult health professional. May perform small sessions throughout the day.

Intensity: Depends on situation, but if weak, ill or convalescing, begin very light to fairly light (RPE 9-11) initially; increasing as tolerated and as advised by a health professional. Do a range of motion only (no bands) if post-surgery, not well-tolerated and/or not medically advised.

Repetitions: Variable depending on tolerance; up to 10-15 (unless otherwise advised).

Sets: 1 set initially; increasing gradually to 2 or 3 as tolerated (unless otherwise advised).

Progression: very slow, based on tolerance (Chapter 2).

Special: For best results, combine with "Basic Stretching Program: In Bed" (Chapter 5).

This program is especially designed for:

- People confined to a bed (temporarily or long-term) for whom exercise would not be dangerous, nor in any way interfere with medical treatment. Discuss with a physician.
- People who may experience postural hypotension (a drop in blood pressure when moving into a sitting or standing position), as can happen in people with chronic fatigue syndrome (Chapter 2)
- People who prefer to do exercise in bed
- People incorporating variety in their program

Please review specific guidelines in Part One.

Note: Be sure to spend a few minutes warming up in bed, moving limbs and muscles in a light, rhythmic fashion, such as "walking in place" horizontally.

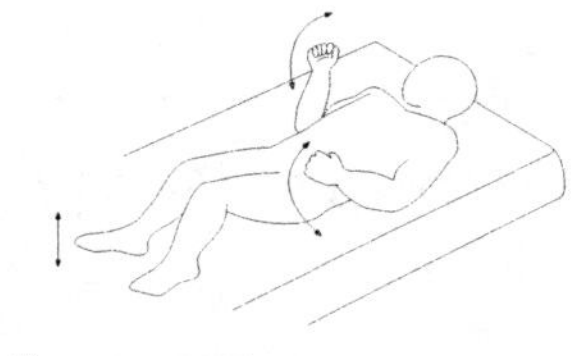

Figure 4-59

Straight Leg Raise

Purpose: Strengthens quadriceps (front of thigh) and hip flexors (top of front of thigh).

Instructions: Lie in bed on your back. Raise one leg toward the ceiling, keeping your knee straight. Slowly lower your back to the bed. Maintain neutral lower-back curve. You may want to position your hands at the lower back to support curve. Repeat.

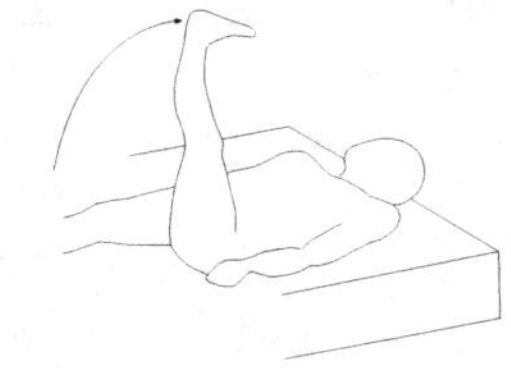

Figure 4-60

Abdominal Squeeze

Purpose: Strengthens abdominal muscles.

Instructions: Lie in bed on your back. Bend both knees. Place your hands on thighs. Push hands on your thighs as hard as possible, while pulling "belly button" toward your spine. Hold for two to five seconds. Do not hold your breath. Repeat.

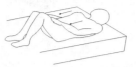

Figure 4-61

Leg Extension

Purpose: Strengthens quadriceps (front of thigh).

Instructions: Lie in bed on your back. Bend both knees. Support one thigh with hands. Extend lower leg until knee is straight, keeping the thigh motionless. You can do this exercise with or without the band, depending on ability. Return to the start position and repeat.

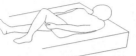
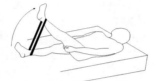

Figure 4-62. Without band

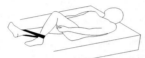

Figure 4-63. With band

Leg Curl

Purpose: Strengthens hamstrings (back of thigh).

Instructions: Lie in bed on your back with both legs straight. Press the heel of one foot into bed and slowly "drag" that foot toward hip, pressing heel continuously against bed. Passively return foot to starting position. Return to the start position and repeat.

Note: For added resistance, anchor a band to the foot of the bed and loop around ankle. Perform as as shown in Figure 4-65.

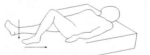

Figure 4-64. Without band

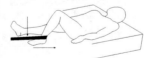

Figure 4-65. With band

Chest Press

Purpose: Strengthens triceps (back of upper arm), pectorals (chest), and deltoids (shoulders).

Instructions: Lie in bed on your back. Grasp one end of the band, and position your hand on your chest. Grasp the band with your other hand 6 to

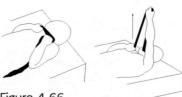

Figure 4-66

12 inches from the first hand. Extend the second hand fully toward the ceiling, keeping the first hand against your chest. Return to the start position and repeat.

Upright Row

Purpose: Strengthens deltoids (top of shoulder) and biceps (front of upper arm).

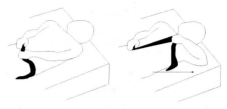

Figure 4-67

Instructions: Lie in bed on your back. Grasp one end of band, and position down by your hips with your arm straight. Grasp band with the other hand 6 to 12 inches from the first hand. Bring the second hand to chin, leading with the elbow and keeping the first hand against your hip. Return to the start position and repeat.

Biceps Curls

Purpose: Strengthens biceps (front of upper arm).

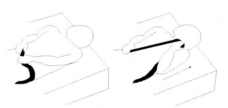

Figure 4-68

Instructions: Lie in bed on your back. Grasp one end of the band and position down by your hips with arm straight. Grasp band with the other hand 6 to 12 inches from first hand. Fully flex the second hand, rotating palm to face your shoulder. Keep the first hand against your hip. Repeat.

Triceps Extensions

Purpose: Strengthens triceps (back of upper arm).

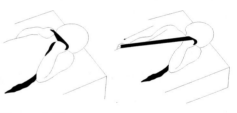

Figure 4-69

Instructions: Lie in bed on your back. Grasp one end of the band, and position against your chin with your arm fully flexed. Grasp band with your other hand 6 to 12 inches from first hand. Fully extend the second hand, keeping the first hand against your chin. Return to the start position and repeat.

Frontal Raise

Purpose: Strengthens deltoids (top of shoulder).

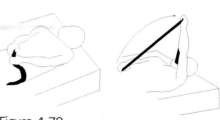

Figure 4-70

Instructions: Lie in bed on your back. Grasp one end of the band and position down by your hips with the arm straight. Grasp band with the other hand 6 to 12 inches from first hand. With palm facing the bed, elevate the second hand toward the ceiling, keeping your elbow straight. Keep the first hand against your hip. Return to the start position and repeat.

Ankle Rotations

Purpose: Strengthens lower leg muscles, maintains pliability of ankles.

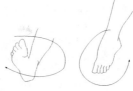

Figure 4-71

Instructions: Lift one foot a few inches off the bed. Draw circles with the foot, first in one direction, and then in the other. Repeat on the other foot.

Wrist Back-and-Forth

Purpose: Strengthens forearms, maintains pliability of wrists.

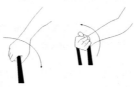

Figure 4-72

Instructions: Grasp band with one hand. Grasp band about 6 to 12 inches away with the other hand. Rotate your wrist back and forth against resistance.

Target Strengthening for the Abdominals

The following is a collection of all the abdominal exercises that appear throughout the book, plus a few more. I get more requests for abdominal exercises than any other single area. "How can I get rid of this?" they say as they pat their middle, wistful expressions on their face. Of course, no one exercise will "get rid of" a wide abdominal girth, and unfortunately, a tendency for excess fat to drift to the mid-section comes with aging. An overall balanced exercise program can help reduce the abdominal girth, and a few abdominal strengthening exercises will at least give the abdominal muscles the shape they are meant to have. More importantly, strong abdominal muscles will help support the spine, and provide support against gravity. That said, it seems everyone just wants that flat profile.

Frequency: 2-3 times per week on nonconsecutive days (unless otherwise advised).

Intensity: Low to moderate (RPE 11-13) initially, gradually progress to moderate to hard (RPE 13-15) as tolerated (unless otherwise advised).

Repetitions: 10-15 (unless otherwise advised).

Sets: 1 set initially, increasing gradually to 2-3 if tolerated (unless otherwise advised).

Rest Periods: 1-2 minutes between sets, unless otherwise advised (Chapter 2).

Progression: Every 2-4 weeks, or longer based on tolerance; no more than 2-5 percent at a time (Chapter 2).

This program is especially designed for:

- People who have a tendency toward back pain
- People who want to improve their abdominal strength
- People seeking a way to combat an expanding waistline (these exercises will provide limited success)

Abdominal Squeeze

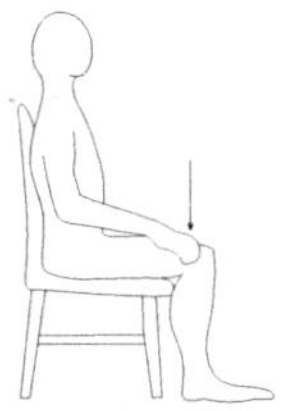

Purpose: Improves strength of abdominal muscles to help stabilize spine.

Instructions: Sit in a chair. Place your hands on your thighs near the knees. Push down firmly on the thighs while tightening the abdominal muscles. Maintain neutral lower-back curve. Hold for three to five seconds. Repeat.

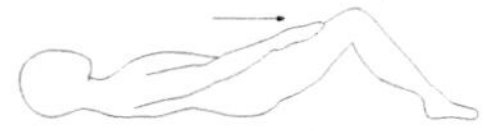

Figure 4-73

Note: This exercise can also be done lying on the floor or bed with knees bent.

Figure 4-74. Lying down

Variation: Repeat previous directions, but place both hands on one thigh near the knee, while turning opposite shoulder toward hands. Hold for three to five seconds. Repeat. Note: This exercise can also be done lying on the floor or bed with knees bent.

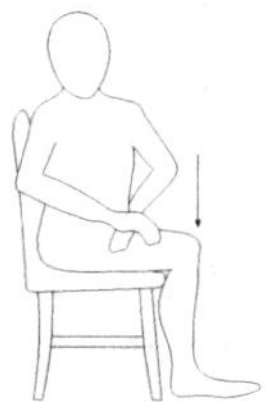

Caution: Avoid overtwisting.

Figure 4-75. Variation

Abdominal Curls

Purpose: Strengthens abdominal muscles.

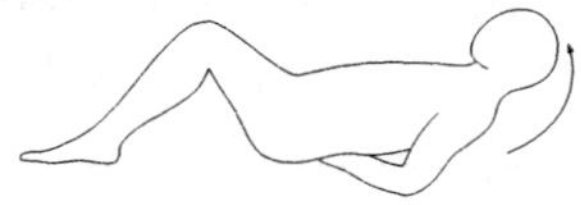

Instructions: Lay on your back on a firm surface. Bend your knees. Place your hands under the lower back to stabilize your pelvis and maintain a neutral spine. Raise your head and shoulders off the

Figure 4-77

ground. Return to the start position and repeat. For more resistance, you may hold a hand weight or other easily managed load against the chest. Be sure to maintain neutral lower-back curve as hands will be holding weight.

Variations:

Keep one leg straight to help maintain neutral lower-back curve.

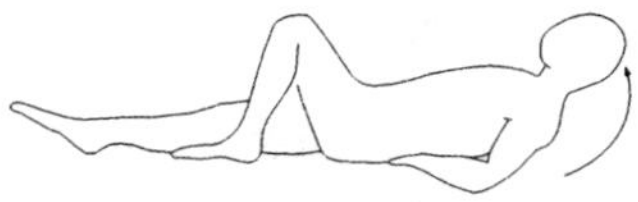

To promote abdominal strength and endurance with variation, do the same as before, only curl to the right, then curl to left (not pictured, see Abdominal Curl illustration for reference).

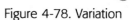

Figure 4-78. Variation

Abdominal Leg Extension

Purpose: Strengthens abdominals.

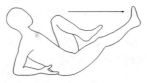

Figure 4-79

Instructions: Lie on the floor on your back. Prop your upper body on your elbows, keeping your head in alignment with spine and placing your hands at the lower back to maintain neutral lower-back curve. If this position is difficult, lie flat on the floor. Pull both knees toward your chest. Extend one knee out to a 45-degree angle. Pull the knee back in and repeat on other side. If abdominal muscles will not support this position, extend the leg higher in air. If any pain or strain is felt in the back, do not do this exercise.

Seated Abdominals

Purpose: Strengthens abdominals.

Instructions:

Preferred method: Choose a chair that has a handle at the top of the chair back. Sit in the chair with good posture. Thread the band through the handle and bring the band over each shoulder. The band should be taut. Bending from the hips, lean torso over thighs. Return to the start.

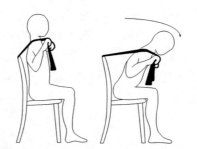

Figure 4-80. Preferred method: band over the shoulders (anchor required)

Alternative method: If chair has no handle, position band across chair back and tuck band under each underarm. The band should be taut. Bending from the hips, lean torso over thighs. Return to the start position and repeat.

Note: You can often use greater resistance on this exercise. Try doubling band or combining two bands together. Use caution with forward flexion with osteoporosis.

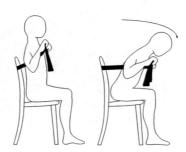

Figure 4-81. Alternative method: band under arms (band across back of chair)

Overhead Abdominal Crunches

Purpose: Strengthens abdominals/internal and external obliques.

Instructions: Anchor middle of the band to a secure overhead hook or bar (a bicycle hook or chin-up bar works well). You may also tie a knot in the center of the band and shut the knot on the other side of the top of the door. Sit in the chair with good posture, positioned directly below the anchor. Grasp ends of the band in each hand, and bring hands to your shoulders, palms facing out. Keeping hands at your shoulders, "shorten" your torso by tightening abdominal muscles and bringing chest closer to thighs.

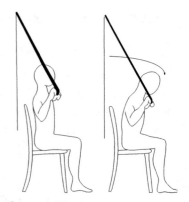

Figure 4-82

Variation: Rotate toward the right thigh; rotate toward the left thigh.

Rotary Torso

Purpose: Strengthens abdominals/internal and external obliques.

Instructions: Sit in a chair. Anchor a band around one arm of the chair, or, if the chair has no arm, around the outermost side bar of chair back. Sit with good posture. Rotate your torso toward the band, being careful not to overtwist. Grasp band with both hands about six inches from chair frame. Using abdominal muscles (not hands), rotate torso to forward facing position. Return to the start position and repeat.

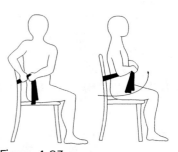

Figure 4-83

Side Bends

Purpose: Strengthens lateral (side) abdominals.

Instructions: Stand with one or both feet on the band (both feet provides more resistance). Grasp ends of the band in each hand, picking up extra slack. With hands by your sides, bend torso to the side. Keep the arms straight, and do not twist. Return to the start position and repeat.

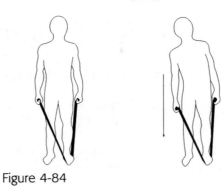

Figure 4-84

Side Bridge

Purpose: Strengthens lateral (side) abdominal with minimal stress on the spine.

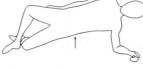

Figure 4-85

Instructions: Lie on your side on the floor. Rest your upper body on your elbow and lower body on your hip. Maintain neutral lower-back curve. With your body straight, lift your hip off the floor so the lower body is resting on your knees. Hold for two to five seconds. Return to the start position and repeat.

Advanced variation: Do the same as previously shown, only lift hip and knees off floor, so lower body is resting on your feet. Do this variation only if you have developed adequate strength from doing the modified side bridge.

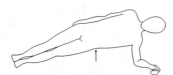

Figure 4-86. Advanced variation

Target Strengthening for the Back

Frequency: Daily (unless otherwise advised).

Intensity: Fairly light (RPE 11) initially, increasing to somewhat hard (RPE 12-13) as tolerated (unless otherwise advised).

Repetitions: 10-15 (unless otherwise advised, see notes that follow and review Lower Back Pain Syndrome in specific conditions section, Chapter 2).

Sets: 1 set (unless otherwise advised).

Special: For best results, combine with Target Stretches for the Back, (Chapter 5).

This program is especially designed for:

- People beginning a post-injury program
- People at risk for injuring their back

The following guidelines come from the extensive research and knowledge of back expert Stuart McGill (2001):

Guidelines for back care:

- Always maintain the natural curves of the spine.
- The popular "pelvic tilt," often used in back exercises, is not recommended, as no evidence suggests that it prevents injury during lifting or exertion and can actually increase the load on the spine.
- Aerobic exercise, such as walking, is one of the best activities to both treat as well as reduce the risk of lower-back injury, especially first-time back injury.
- Contrary to popular belief, most back flexibility exercises do not improve back health nor lessen risk of injury. Greater flexibility at hips and knees does seem to provide benefit.
- Back flexibility should not be emphasized when the back is injured until spine is "stabilized" and has been conditioned with strength and endurance exercise. In particular, reduce injury risk by avoiding full-range spine motion in the morning after rising from bed when discs are more hydrated.
- No single exercise is best for the abdominal muscles, as no exercise utilizes all the abdominal muscles. The best to start with would be variations of the curl-up (with lower back supported) and isometric side bridge (see Figures 4-92 and 4-93).

- Do not emphasize strength (using high intensity) in lower-back exercises. Rather, do more repetitions of less demanding exercises to enhance both endurance and strength. (e.g., lower intensity/higher repetitions).
- Most popular back-extension exercises place a high load on the spine (such as lying facedown on the floor and raising the upper body and legs off the floor). Modified single leg extension hold, as pictured in Figure 4-90, minimizes load on the spine.
- Have patience, and be compliant. Reduced pain and better function may not occur for up to three months.

The following exercises are not the best suited for every individual. Rather, they have been formally evaluated (McGill, 2001) and have been selected for minimizing load on the spine and based on knowledge of how back injuries occur. More fit people can tolerate greater load levels.

Slow Lunges

Purpose: Promotes hip and knee mobility, muscle strength, and muscle endurance.

Instructions: Stand with one foot in front of the other. Keep torso upright at all times, maintaining neutral lower-back curve. Slowly lunge forward, bending the front knee no greater than a 90-degree angle. Switch legs after each repetition.

Figure 4-87

Abdominal Curls

Purpose: Strengthens abdominal muscles.

Figure 4-88

Instructions: Lay on your back on a firm surface. Bend the knees. Place your hands under the lower back to stabilize pelvis and maintain a neutral spine. Raise your head and shoulders off the ground. Return to the start position and repeat. For more resistance, you may hold a hand weight or other easily managed load against the chest. Be sure to maintain neutral lower-back curve as hands will be holding weight.

Variation: Keep one leg straight to help maintain neutral lower-back curve.

Figure 4-89

Alternating Abdominal Curls

Purpose: Promotes abdominal strength and endurance with variation.

Instructions: Do the same as previously shown, only curl to the right, return to the start position, and then curl to left. Repeat. (not pictured, see Abdominal Curl illustration for reference).

Single-Leg Extension Hold

Purpose: Promotes the strength and endurance of spine muscles while minimizing the load on the spine.

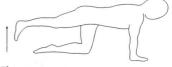

Figure 4-90

Instructions: Get on your hands and knees. Maintain neutral lower-back curve. Extend one leg straight back with your toes resting on the floor. Slowly raise your leg no more than parallel to the floor. Hold for two to five seconds. Return to the start position and repeat.

Advanced variation: Reaching forward with the opposite arm increases muscle activity, but also adds load on your spine. Do not do this exercise if your back is injured or if you are in the beginning stages of back exercises.

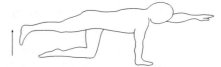

Figure 4-91. Advanced variation

Side Bridge

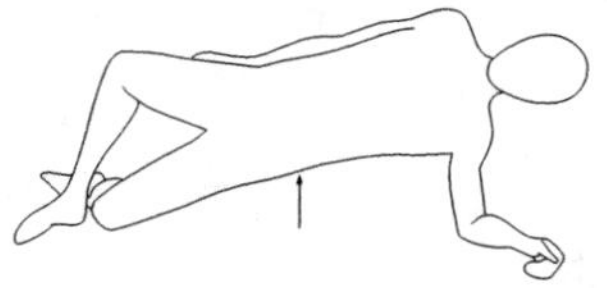

Purpose: Strengthens lateral (side) abdominal with minimal stress on the spine.

Instructions: Lie on your side on the floor. Rest your upper body on your elbow and lower body on your hip. Maintain neutral lower-back curve. With your body straight, lift your hip off the floor so your lower body is resting on your knees. Hold for two to five seconds. Return to the start position and repeat.

Figure 4-92

Advanced variation: Do the same as previously shown, only lift the hip and knees off floor, so the lower body is resting on your feet. Do this variation only if you have developed adequate strength from doing the modified side bridge.

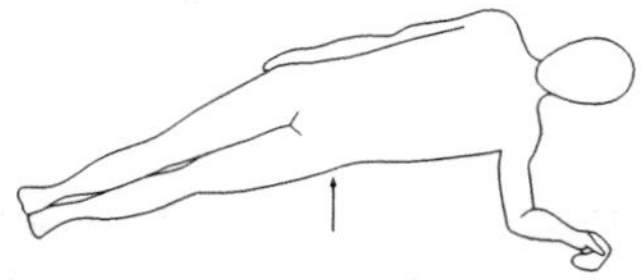

Figure 4-93. Advanced variation

Target Strengthening for the Hips, Knees, and Ankles

Frequency: 2-3 times per week on nonconsecutive days (unless otherwise advised).

Intensity: Low to moderate (RPE 11-13) initially, especially if area is painful, weak, and/or unstable. Gradually progress to moderate to hard (RPE 13-15) as tolerated (unless otherwise advised). If post-surgery, do not add additional resistance until you are 6 weeks post-surgery and you have your doctor's permission.

Repetitions: 10-15 if for rehab or over 60 years old; 8-12 if healthy and under 60 years old (unless otherwise advised).

Sets: 1 set initially; increasing gradually to 2-3 if tolerated (unless otherwise advised).

Rest Periods: 1-2 minutes between sets, unless otherwise advised (Chapter 2).

Progression: every 2-4 weeks, or longer based on tolerance; no more than 2-10 percent at a time (Chapter 2).

Selections: Choose exercises specific to your area of concern that you can tolerate relatively pain-free. The intention is not for you to do all the following exercises. For best results, incorporate a few of the most appropriate exercises into one of the basic programs, making substitutions so that no more than a total of 12 exercises are performed.

Combinations of these target exercises are appropriate for:

- *Balance problems:* Choose a couple from each area and vary routinely.
- *Hip or knee replacements:* Strengthen muscles around replaced joint.
- *Peripheral artery disease (reduced blood flow) in legs:* See the following group of exercises, Target Strengthening for Peripheral Arterial Disease in this chapter.
- *Arthritis:* Choose exercises around painful joints that are well tolerated.
- Anyone interested in further strengthening/stabilizing in these areas

HIPS

Note: The following three exercises (hip extension, abduction, and adduction) can be easily performed as a group. Simply get into position with the band around one ankle and attached to a secure anchor, and rotate as you do all three in sequence on one side. Repeat all three exercises in sequence on other leg.

Hip Extension

Purpose: Strengthens gluteal muscles (buttocks).

Instructions: Tie the band in a loop. Place one end of the loop round a secure anchor at ankle height. Place other end of the loop around ankle. Stand next to a secure support (wall, table, chair, etc.). Keeping the knee straight and toes pointing forward, lift one heel behind you. Do not rotate your hips to the side. Return to the start position and repeat.

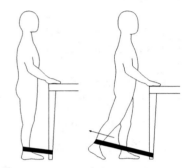

Figure 4-94

Hip Abduction

Purpose: Strengthens gluteus medius (side of hip).

Instructions: Tie the band in a loop. Place one end of the loop around a secure anchor at ankle height (can also use opposite ankle as anchor). Place other end of the loop around ankle furthest from the anchor. Stand next to an anchor secure support (wall, table, chair, etc.). Keeping the knee straight and toes pointing forward, move the leg away from midline of the body. Return to the start position and repeat.

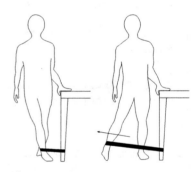

Figure 4-95

Note: This exercise can also be done sitting (as pictured) or lying on side (not pictured). Return to the start position and repeat.

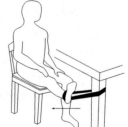

Figure 4-96

Hip Adduction

Purpose: Strengthens inner thigh muscles; also good for knee stability.

Instructions: Stand next to a secure support (wall, table, chair, etc.). Tie the band in a loop. Place one end of the loop around the secure anchor at ankle height. Place the other end of the loop around the ankle that is nearest to the anchor. Keeping knee straight and toes pointing forward, move leg toward midline of body. Return to the start position and repeat.

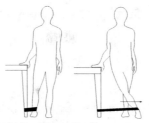

Figure 4-97

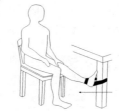

Figure 4-98

Stepping

Purpose: Strengthens primarily quadriceps (front of upper thigh) and gluteals (buttocks).

Instructions: Step up and down on a bench or stair, starting with low step if necessary (four inches) and increasing to 10 to 12 inches as tolerated. Use same lead leg for 8 to 12 reps. Switch and repeat on other leg.

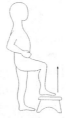

Figure 4-99

Note: Avoid this exercise or minimize step height if it aggravates your knees or hips. If you are ready for more resistance, hold a progressively larger hand weight in each hand as you step.

KNEES

Thigh Squeeze

Purpose: Strengthens quadriceps (front of thigh).

Instructions: Sit with hips toward front of the chair. Extend one leg straight in front of you, with toes pointing up and your heel resting on the floor. Tighten the thigh muscle of the extended leg. Hold for three to five seconds. Repeat.

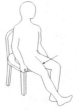

Figure 4-100

Note: This exercise can also be done sitting on the floor or in bed.

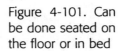

Figure 4-101. Can be done seated on the floor or in bed

Straight Leg Raise #1

Purpose: Strengthens quadriceps (front of thigh).

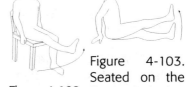

Instructions: Sit with your hips toward the front of the chair. Extend one leg straight in front of you, with toes pointing up and your heel resting on the floor. Keeping knee straight, raise extended leg to parallel to floor. Hold for three to five seconds. Return to the start position and repeat.

Figure 4-102   Figure 4-103. Seated on the floor or in bed

Note: This exercise can also be done sitting on the floor or in bed.

Straight Leg Raise #2

Purpose: Strengthens quadriceps (front of thigh).

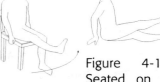

Instructions: Sit with your hips toward the front of the chair. Extend one leg straight in front of you, with toes pointing up and your heel resting on the Floor. Keeping knee straight, perform as in Figure 4-102, raising extended leg to parallel to floor, but don't hold. Return to the start position and repeat.

Figure 4-104   Figure 4-105. Seated on the floor or in bed

Note: This exercise can also be done sitting on the floor or in bed.

Terminal Extensions

Purpose: Focuses on "vastus medialis" (innermost muscle) of quadriceps (front of thigh).

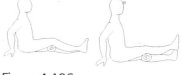

Figure 4-106

Instructions: Sit in a chair, in bed, or on the floor with leg(s) straight in front of you. Flex knee of one leg 10 to 15 degrees. (If on the floor or in bed, put rolled up towel or cushion under knee). Straighten the leg. Hold for three to five seconds. Return to the start position and repeat.

Leg Extension

Purpose: Strengthens quadriceps (front of thigh).

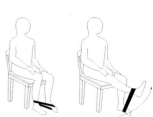

Instructions: Tie the band in a loop. Step on the band with one foot and loop *around* the other ankle (leg you will use first). Stabilize the thigh by tucking both hands under it. Sit with both legs at 90-degree angle. Fully straighten the leg; pausing at full extension. Return to the start position and repeat.

Figure 4-107

Hamstring Curl

Purpose: Strengthens hamstrings (back of thigh).

Instructions: Stand behind a chair or next to support. Tie the band in a loop. Stand on the loop with one leg, position band around the other ankle. Bending knee, pull the heel toward hip to 90-degree angle. Keep the knee pointing toward the floor. Avoid allowing the knee to "pull forward." Return to the start position and repeat.

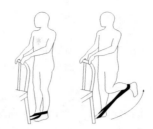

Figure 4-108

ANKLE

Calf Raises

Purpose: Strengthens calf muscles.

Instructions: Stand on a stair with the ball of your foot on the edge of the stair. Allow the heels to drop below the edge of the stair, so that the heels are lower than the toes. Rise up on the toes as much as possible. You can do both feet at a time or one foot at a time. Return to the start position and repeat.

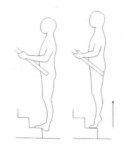

Figure 4-109

Variations: After completing set with toes pointing straight forward, perform one set with toes pointing in, then one with toes pointing out. You can perform the toe push sitting in a chair with an elastic band as shown in Figure 4-110.

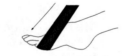

Figure 4-110. Variation

Toe Pull

Purpose: Strengthens shin muscles.

Instructions: Tie the band in a loop. Attach one end to a secure anchor at ankle/knee height. Sit in a chair. Position the other end of loop across the top of your foot. Start with toes forward, while not allowing band to slip off foot. Pull toes toward you. Return to the start position and repeat.

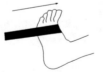

Figure 4-111

Ankle Range of Motion Series

❏Ankle Rotations

Purpose: Strengthens lower leg muscles; improves pliability of ankle joint.

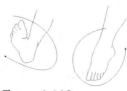

Figure 4-112

Instructions: Lift one foot a few inches off the floor. Draw circles with the foot, first in one direction, then in the other. Repeat on the other leg.

❏"Happy feet" (Inversion/Eversion)

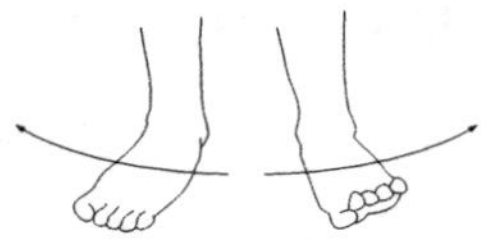

Purpose: Strengthens lower leg muscles; improves pliability of ankle joint.

Figure 4-113

Instructions: Lift one foot a few inches off the floor. Draw a "smile" (half-circle) with the foot in both directions. Repeat on other leg.

❏Toe point/flex

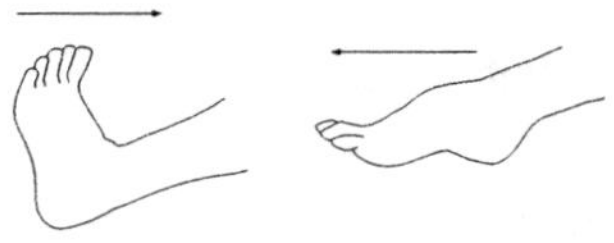

Purpose: Strengthens lower leg muscles; improves pliability of ankle joint.

Instructions: Lift one foot a few inches off the floor. Push toes forward, and then pull back. Repeat on the other leg.

Figure 4-114

Target Strengthening for the Shoulders

Frequency: 2-3 times per week on nonconsecutive days (unless otherwise advised).

Intensity: If post-surgery, very light to fairly light (RPE 9-11), otherwise, low to moderate initially (RPE 11-13), especially if area is painful, weak, and/or unstable. Gradually progress to moderate to hard (RPE 13-15) as tolerated (unless otherwise advised). If post-surgery, do not add additional resistance until you are 6 weeks post-surgery and you have your doctor's permission.

Repetitions: 10-15 if for rehab or over 60 years old; 8-12 if healthy and under 60 years of age (unless otherwise advised).

Sets: 1 set initially; increasing gradually to 2-3 if tolerated (unless otherwise advised).

Rest Periods: 1-2 minutes between sets, unless otherwise advised (Chapter 2).

Progression: Every 2-4 weeks, or longer based on tolerance; no more than 2-5 percent at a time, since it is an area involving smaller muscle groups (Chapter 2).

Selections: Choose exercises specific to your area of concern that you can tolerate relatively pain-free. The intention is not for you to do all the exercises listed. For best results, incorporate a few of the most appropriate exercises below into one of the basic programs, making substitutions so that not more than a total of 12 exercises are performed.

Combinations of these target exercises are appropriate for:

- *Shoulder issues/instability:* Rotary cuff, bursitis, tendonitis, arthritis, or otherwise unstable shoulder joint

- Anyone interested in further strengthening/stabilizing the shoulder area

- See the following set of exercises in this chapter: Target Strengthening for Post-Breast Cancer or Chest Surgery. Many of these exercises are also appropriate for shoulder rehabilitation/stabilization.

Bent-Over Row

Purpose: Strengthens biceps (front of upper arm) and upper-back muscles, stabilizes shoulder joint.

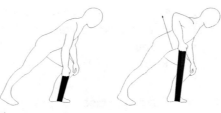

Instructions: Grasp the end of the band in each hand. Step on the middle of the band. Bend the torso forward and

Figure 4-115

rest your hand (on same side as forward leg) on your knee for support (can also use the back of a chair, counter, or table for support instead of the knee). Straighten other arm toward the floor. Take excess slack out of the band as needed. Pull your elbow (not hand) toward the ceiling in full flexion. Return to the start position and repeat.

Note: Be sure your upper body is supported to protect your back. Use caution with forward flexion with osteoporosis.

Shoulder Diagonal Sweep High to Low

Purpose: Strengthens front of shoulder and chest muscles, helps stabilize shoulder joint.

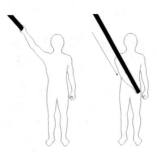

Instructions: Anchor band above shoulder height. Stand with your side to the band. With the arm nearest the band, grasp the band at shoulder level. Sweep arm diagonally down across the body, ending with the arm low across the body and the palm facing behind you. Return to the start position and repeat.

Figure 4-116

Shoulder Cross Diagonal Sweep High to Low

Purpose: Strengthens back of shoulder and upper-back muscles, helps stabilize shoulder joint.

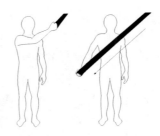

Instructions: Anchor band above shoulder height. Stand with your side to the band. With your outside arm, cross your body, reaching up to grasp the band at shoulder level. Sweep your arm diagonally down

Figure 4-117

across your body, ending with the arm at your side, the elbow straight, and the palm facing out. Return to the start position and repeat.

Shoulder Cross Diagonal Sweep Low to High

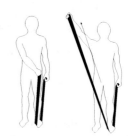

Purpose: Strengthens back of shoulder and upper-back muscles, helps stabilize shoulder joint.

Instructions: Anchor band below shoulder height (can also anchor with foot, as shown in Figure 4-118). Stand with your side to the band. With your outside arm, cross your body, reaching down to grasp the band at hip level. Sweep your arm diagonally up across your body, ending up with arm high, elbow slightly flexed, and palm facing out.

Figure 4-118

Rotary Cuff Exercise Series

❏ Rotary Cuff #1

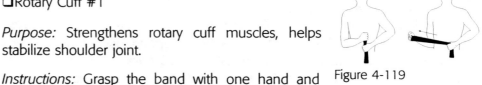

Purpose: Strengthens rotary cuff muscles, helps stabilize shoulder joint.

Instructions: Grasp the band with one hand and anchor to one side at waist level. Reach across your body with the other arm and grasp the band, keeping elbow tucked against body. Rotate your forearm horizontally across your body, without moving the upper arm or the anchor arm.

Figure 4-119

❏ Rotary Cuff #2

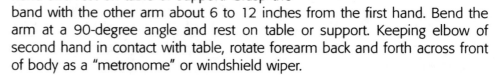

Purpose: Strengthens rotary cuff muscles, helps stabilize shoulder joint.

Instructions: Grasp on end of the band with hand and rest on table or support. Grasp the band with the other arm about 6 to 12 inches from the first hand. Bend the arm at a 90-degree angle and rest on table or support. Keeping elbow of second hand in contact with table, rotate forearm back and forth across front of body as a "metronome" or windshield wiper.

Figure 4-120

❏ Rotary Cuff #3

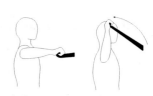

Purpose: Strengthens rotary cuff muscles, helps stabilize shoulder joint.

Instructions: Anchor band at chest level by attaching to hook, bar, or tying a knot in band and shutting on the other side of a door. Position body facing the anchor. Bend the arm at a 90-degree angle, upper arm pointing out to the side (and upper arm parallel

Figure 4-121

to the floor) and forearm pointing toward the anchor. Grasp the band near the anchor and rotate the forearm up toward the ceiling and back toward the anchor as a "metronome."

Target Strengthening for Post-Breast Cancer or Chest Surgery

Frequency: 2-3 times/week (unless otherwise advised).

Intensity: If post-surgery, should be very light to fairly light (RPE 9-11). Otherwise, fairly light (RPE 11) initially; increasing to somewhat hard (RPE 12-13) as tolerated (unless otherwise advised). If post-surgery, do not add additional resistance until you are 6 weeks post-surgery and you have your doctor's permission.

Repetitions: Work up to 8-12 (unless otherwise advised). You do not need to complete all the exercises in the beginning.

Sets: 1 set initially (unless otherwise advised); progress to 2-3 as tolerated.

Rest Periods: 1-2 minutes between sets, unless otherwise advised (Chapter 2).

Selections: The intention is not for you to do all the exercises listed to start with. Do a few, and work up to being able to do them all. These exercises focus on range of motion, preparing postural and upper body for more strenuous loads.

Progression: If you can complete these exercises with no negative signs/symptoms (including swelling, numbness, redness, achyness, change in tissue texture), and if you have regained full range of motion on your affected side (in the case of breast cancer surgery), you are probably ready for more resistance (Chapter 2).

Special:

If you have had breast cancer surgery:

- Watch for signs of swelling and pain in your affected arm. Don't push through achiness or heaviness.
- Focus on regaining full range of motion on your affected side.

If you have had open heart surgery:

- Watch for signs of the sternum healing. You should experience no sense of movement or sound of clicking or popping

Combinations of these target exercises are also appropriate for:

- Chest surgery: open heart surgery, lung volume reduction, heart transplant, lung transplant

- Shoulder issues/instability: Rotary cuff, bursitis, tendonitis, arthritis, or otherwise unstable shoulder joint. You can combine some of these exercises with previous group of exercises in this chapter, Target Strengthening for the Shoulders.

- Anyone interested in further strengthening/stabilizing the shoulder and chest area

Abdominal Strengthener

Purpose: Begins to strengthen the abdominal muscles, which help stabilize the spine. This exercise focuses on the transverse abdominal muscle, which lies below the top layer of abdominal muscle. As this muscle remains intact when a TRAM flap (mastectomy procedure) is performed, this exercise is safe after surgery.

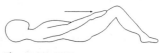

Figure 4-122

Instructions: Start gently, but as soon after surgery as possible (check with your surgeon first). You may be more comfortable starting this exercise in a lying down position. Do not bear down or push abdominal muscles out. Lie on your back with the knees bent. First, pull the abdomen in toward spine—"belly button to backbone"—while maintaining the neutral lower-back curve. Second, pull abdominal muscles in even more, pressing spine on the floor. Hold for 10 seconds. Repeat.

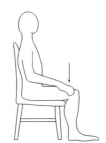

Figure   4-123. Seated

Note: This exercise can also be done sitting or standing, and you can repeat it several times per day.

Hand Lean

Purpose: Begins to strengthen the muscles in chest and shoulder.

Instructions: Sit on a bed or the floor with the palm of the affected arm down alongside you. Lean some of your body weight on your hand. Over time, increase the amount of weight as you lean. Vary the position of the hand (e.g., farther away from your body) behind you, out to the side. Increase the amount of weight in these different positions over time. Hold for 10 seconds in each position.

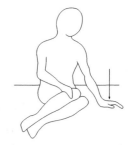

Figure 4-124. Seated

Lateral Raise

Purpose: Begins to strengthen the muscles used for shoulder abduction (moving arms away from body).

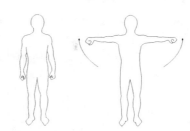

Figure 4-125

Instructions: Stand with your feet shoulder-width apart and arms hanging at sides. Raise your arms out to your sides until parallel to floor, palms facing the floor. Return to the start position and repeat.

Advanced: When at least 6 weeks post-surgery and/or with physicians permission, you may add low resistance using a band (i.e., tan or yellow).

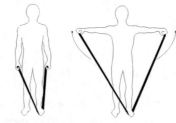

Figure 4-126

Frontal Raise

Purpose: Begins to strengthen the deltoid muscles for shoulder flexion.

Instructions: Position arms at sides, palms facing behind you. Slowly raise arms in front of you to parallel to the floor, or as high as affected arm will let you reach. Return to the start position and repeat.

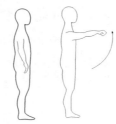

Figure 4-127

Advanced: When at least six weeks post-surgery and/or with physicians permission, you may add low resistance using a band (i.e., tan or yellow).

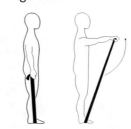

Figure 4-128

Biceps Curl

Purpose: Begins to strengthen the muscles in front of upper arm.

Instructions: Position arms at sides. Face thumb side of hand forward and close hands in loose grip. Keeping elbows "glued to ribs" and shoulder blades down and back, slowly raise your hands toward your shoulders. Return to the start position and repeat.

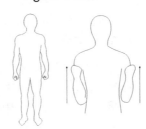

Figure 4-129

Advanced: When at least six weeks post-surgery and/or with physicians permission, you may add low resistance using a band (i.e., tan or yellow).

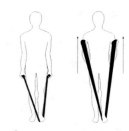

Figure   4-130.
Advanced: with band

Shoulder Extension

Purpose: Begins to strengthen the muscles in the upper back and triceps (back of upper arm).

Instructions: Position your arms at your sides, palms facing behind you. Keeping shoulders down and back and chest lifted, raise your arms behind you, keeping the elbows straight. Return to the start position and repeat.

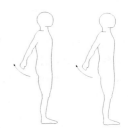

Figure 4-131

Advanced: When at least six weeks post-surgery and/or with physicians permission, you may add low resistance using a band (i.e., tan or yellow).

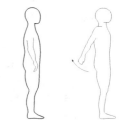

Figure 4-132

Triceps Press

Purpose: Begins to strengthen triceps (back of upper arm).

Instructions: Position your arms at your sides, palms facing your body. Lift your elbows behind you with the arm fully flexed. Slowly straighten your arms. Return to the start, keeping elbows behind you. Return to the start position and repeat.

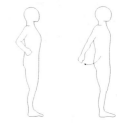

Figure 4-133

Advanced: When at least six weeks post-surgery and/or with physicians permission, you may add low resistance using a band (i.e., tan or yellow).

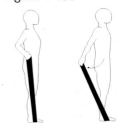

Figure 4-134

Hands and Knees

Purpose: Helps to strengthen the chest and shoulder muscles, and stretches underarm and shoulder.

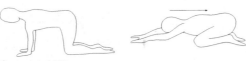

Figure 4-135

Instructions: Position your body on your hands and knees, with your hands directly under your shoulders (fingers facing forward). Keep your arms straight but not locked,you're your head and neck in alignment with your spine. Keep your weight mostly on the knees and the unaffected arm. Keeping your hands planted, slowly move your hips backward and rest buttocks on your heels. Lower your head toward the floor. Hold for five seconds. Return to the start position and repeat.

Serratus Reach

Purpose: Begins to strengthen the serratus anterior muscles that hold shoulder blades against the back.

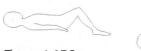

Figure 4-136

Instructions: Lie on your back with your knees bent and your feet flat on the floor. Raise both arms toward the ceiling with palms facing your feet. Keeping your head and back on the floor, lift your shoulders off the floor. Hold for five seconds. Return to the start position and repeat.

Lower-Back Bridge

Purpose: Strengthens muscles of the lower back, hamstrings (back of thigh) and gluteals (buttocks). Especially helpful post-TRAM flap (mastectomy procedure).

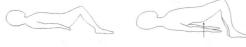

Figure 4-137

Instructions: Lie on your back with your knees bent and your feet flat on the floor. Raise your hips off the floor to form a straight line from your chin to your knees at the same time as you contract the abdominals, lower back, and buttocks. Maintain a neutral lower-back curve. Hold for five seconds. Return to the start position and repeat.

Target Strengthening
for Peripheral Arterial Disease

Frequency: 2-3 times/week (unless otherwise advised).

Intensity: Fairly light (RPE 11) initially; increasing to somewhat hard (RPE 12-13) as tolerated (unless otherwise advised). This level may mean starting some of these exercises without added resistance, (i.e., not using an elastic band). Ultimately, progress to hard (RPE 15).

Repetitions: 8-12 (unless otherwise advised).

Sets: 1 set initially; progress to 2-3 as tolerated.

Rest Periods: 1-2 minutes between sets, unless otherwise advised (Chapter 2).

Progression: Based on tolerance (Chapter 2).

Selections: For best results, supplement these exercises with a combination of upper-body and torso exercises. Refer to one of the basic resistance training programs in this section.

Special: Supplement these resistance training exercises with regular walking, performed at a leg pain of "8" (hard) on the claudication scale (Appendix D).

Stepping

Purpose: Strengthens primarily quadriceps (front of upper thigh) and gluteals (buttocks).

Instructions: Step up and down on a bench or a stair, starting with a low step if necessary (4 inches) and increasing to 10 to 12 inches as tolerated. Return to the start position and repeat. Repeat on the other leg after completing all reps on the first leg. If you are ready for more resistance, hold a progressively larger hand weight in each hand as you step.

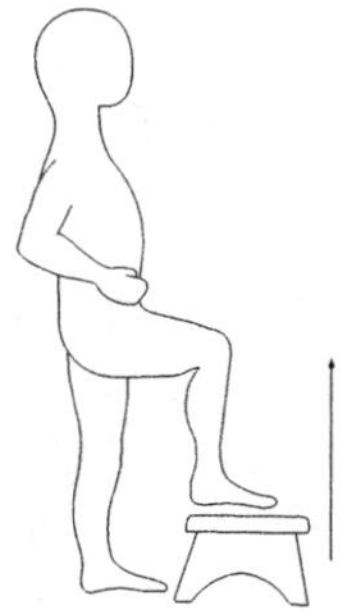

Figure 4-138

Note: Avoid this exercise or minimize step height if it aggravates your knees or hips.

Note: The following three exercises (hip extension, abduction, and adduction) can be easily performed as a group. Simply get into position with the band around one ankle and attached to a secure anchor, and rotate as you do all three in sequence on one side. Repeat all three in sequence on the other leg.

Hip Extension

Purpose: Strengthens gluteal muscles (buttocks).

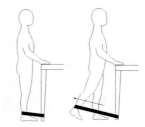

Figure 4-139

Instructions: Tie band in loop. Place one end of loop around a secure anchor at ankle height. Place other end of loop around ankle. Stand next to a secure support (wall, table, chair, etc.). Keeping knee straight and toes pointing forward, lift one heel behind you. Do not rotate your hips to the side. Return to the start position and repeat.

Hip Abduction

Purpose: Strengthens gluteus medius (side of hip).

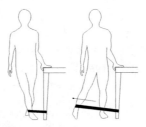

Figure 4-140

Instructions: Tie a band in a loop. Place one end of the loop around a secure anchor at ankle height (can also use opposite ankle as anchor). Place other end of the loop around ankle *furthest from anchor*. Stand next to a secure support (wall, table, chair, etc.). Keeping knee straight and toes pointing forward, move the leg *away* from the midline of the body. Return to the start position and repeat.

Note: This exercise can also be done sitting (as pictured in Figure 4-141) or lying on side (not pictured). Return to the start position and repeat.

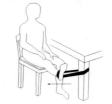

Figure 4-141

Hip Adduction

Purpose: Strengthens inner thigh muscles; also good for knee stability.

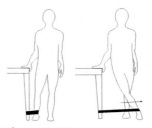

Figure 4-142

Instructions: Tie a band in a loop. Place one end of the loop around secure anchor at ankle height. Place the other end of the loop around the ankle nearest the anchor. Stand next to a secure support (wall, table, chair, etc.). Keeping knee straight and toes pointing forward, move leg *toward* the midline of the body. Return to the start position and repeat.

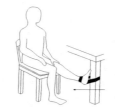

Figure 4-143. Seated

Squats (modified)

Purpose: Strengthens quadriceps and gluteals (buttocks).

Instructions: Step on a band with one foot or two (using both feet adds to resistance load). Pick up slack so that band is taut. Stand with good posture: feet shoulder-width apart or slightly wider, arms straight at your sides. Bend both knees to about a 45-degree angle, or within knee stability range. Weight will be primarily on the balls of your feet. Do not lean your torso forward—remain upright. Return to the start position and repeat.

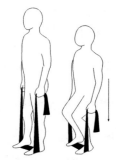

Figure 4-144

Calf Raises (Foot Plantar flexion)

Purpose: Strengthens calf muscles.

Instructions: Stand on a stair with the ball of your foot on the edge of a stair. Allow your heels to drop below the edge of the stair, so that your heels are lower than your toes. Rise up on your toes as much as possible. Return to the start. You can do both at a time or one at a time.

Variation: After completing a set with the toes pointing straight forward, perform one set with the *toes pointing in*, then one with *toes pointing out*.

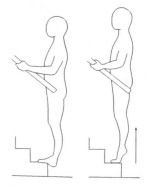

Figure 4-145

Target Strengthening for Osteoporosis

If you have or suspect osteoporosis, consult physician before beginning these exercises.

Frequency: 3 times/week (unless otherwise advised).

Intensity: Begin exercises at low intensity (RPE 10-11), initially, increasing gradually to somewhat hard (RPE 12-13) as tolerated (unless otherwise advised). If you do not yet have osteoporosis (or it is not severe and you are cleared by your physician), and if you have been consistent with your program long term (3-6 months), progress gradually to moderate-high intensity (75-85 percent of maximum; RPE 15).

Repetitions: 8-12 (unless otherwise advised).

Sets: 1 set initially (unless otherwise advised); progress to 3 as tolerated.

Rest Periods: 1-2 minutes between sets, unless otherwise advised (Chapter 2).

Progression: Gradual, based on tolerance and physician recommendations; no more than 2-10 percent increase at a time; the higher end of range for exercises using larger muscle groups and multiple joints; lower end of range for exercises using small muscle groups and single joints (Chapter 2).

Selections: Choose 6-12 exercises listed in this section. Once an initial, symptom-free, consistent base is developed (at least 3 months), vary the exercise selection, including exercises that allow you safely use greater loads. Routinely vary selections and exercise sequence to keep bone from getting too much predictable repetition. Bone likes to be "surprised."

Special: Always use good posture. Be particularly cautious of any forward flexion (leaning forward) movements, always maintaining lower-back curve and bending from hips. When leaning forward, "push buttocks out behind you" rather than rounding spine. Though many of these can be done sitting, they are most effective performed standing, due to force exerted in standing position. Review discussion of Osteoporosis in Chapter 2.

Combinations of these target exercises are appropriate for:

- *Osteoporosis:* People diagnosed with clinically significant bone mineral density loss, usually in spine, hip/thigh, and/or wrist

- *Osteopenia:* People with reduced—but not diagnostic—bone mineral density.

• Risk for osteoporosis/osteopenia: For preventive purposes, be aware of factors that increase risk: women (especially of small stature and/or of advancing age), Caucasian/Asian race, premature menopause or prolonged loss of menstrual periods, low physical activity, chronic smoking, excessive alcohol consumption, low dietary calcium intake, family history, chronic use of medications that promote bone loss (such as corticosteroids).

Stepping

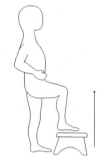

Purpose: Strengthens primarily quadriceps (front of upper thigh) and gluteals (buttocks), focuses on bone in hip area.

Instructions: Step up and down on a bench or stair, starting with low step if necessary (4 inches) and increasing to 10 to 12 inches as tolerated. Return to the start position and repeat. Repeat on other leg after completing all reps on the first leg. If you are ready for more resistance, hold a progressively larger hand weight in each hand as you step.

Figure 4-146

Note: Avoid this exercise or minimize step height if it aggravates your knees or hips.

Note: The following three exercises (hip extension, abduction, and adduction) can be easily performed as a group. Simply get in to position with the band around one ankle and attached to a secure anchor, and rotate as you do all three in sequence on one side. Repeat all three in sequence on other leg.

Hip Extension

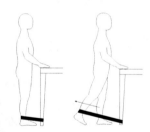

Purpose: Strengthens gluteal muscles (buttocks), focuses on bone in hip area.

Instructions: Tie band in a loop. Place one end of the loop around a secure anchor at ankle height. Place the other end of the loop around the ankle. Stand next to a secure support (wall, table, chair, etc.). Keeping the knee straight and toes pointing forward, lift one heel behind you. Do not rotate the hips to the side. Return to the start position and repeat.

Figure 4-147

Hip Abduction

Purpose: Strengthens gluteus medius (side of hip), focuses on bone in hip area.

Instructions: Tie band in a loop. Place one end of the loop around secure anchor at ankle height (can also use opposite ankle as anchor). Place other end of the loop around the ankle furthest from the anchor. Stand next to a secure support (wall, table, chair, etc.). Keeping the knee straight and toes pointing forward, move the leg away from the midline of the body. Return to the start position and repeat.

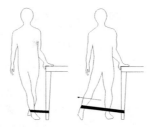

Figure 4-148

Note: This exercise can also be done sitting (as pictured in Figure 4-149) or lying on side (not pictured). Return to the start position and repeat.

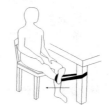

Figure 4-149

Hip Adduction

Purpose: Strengthens inner thigh muscles; also good for knee stability, focuses on bone in hip area.

Instructions: Tie band in a loop. Place one end of the loop around a secure anchor at ankle height. Place the other end of the loop around the ankle nearest the anchor. Stand next to a secure support (wall, table, chair, etc.). Keeping the knee straight and toes pointing forward, move the leg *toward* the midline of the body. Return to the start position and repeat.

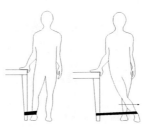

Figure 4-150

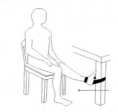

Figure 4-151. Seated

Back Extension

Purpose: Strengthens back muscles; focuses on bone in spine area.

Instructions: Step on band with one foot or two (using both feet adds to resistance load). Grasp end of band in each hand. Pick up slack so that the band is taut. Either stand or remain seated. Lean forward to approximately a 45-degree angle, bending from the hips and maintaining neutral lower-back curve. Keeping elbows straight, carefully erect your torso to upright position. Return to the start position and repeat.

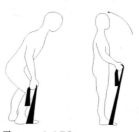

Figure 4-152

Note: It is very important not to round the back when doing this exercise. This exercise can be performed sitting or standing.

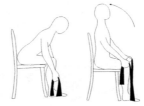

Figure 4-153

Squats (modified)

Purpose: Strengthens quadriceps and gluteals (buttocks), focuses on bone in hip area.

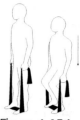

Figure 4-154

Instructions: Step on a band with one foot or two (using both feet adds to resistance load). Pick up the slack so that the band is taut. Stand with good posture: feet shoulder-width apart or slightly wider, arms straight at sides. Bend both knees to about a 45-degree angle, or within knee stability range. Weight will be primarily on the balls of the feet. Do not lean your torso forward—remain upright. Return to the start position and repeat.

Slow Lunges (An Alternative to Squats)

Purpose: Promotes hip and knee mobility, quadriceps strength, focuses on bone in hip area.

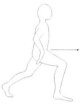

Figure 4-155

Instructions: Stand with one foot in front of the other. Keep your torso upright at all times, maintaining neutral lower-back curve. Slowly lunge forward, bending front knee no greater than 90-degree angle. Switch after each repetition.

Seated Row

Purpose: Strengthens biceps (front of upper arm) and upper back.

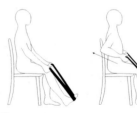

Figure 4-156

Instructions: Sit in chair with one leg extended. Loop the band across the sole of the extended foot. Grasp the band in each hand about 12 inches from the foot on each side, taking up excess slack. Maintain neutral lower-back curve. Pull both elbows straight back to full flexion. Return to the start position and repeat.

Note: This exercise can also be done sitting on the floor or in bed.

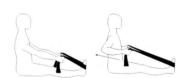

Figure 4-157. Seated on the floor or in bed

Lat Pull-Down

Purpose: Strengthens primarily latissimus dorsi (mid back) and biceps (front of upper arm), focuses on bone in spine area.

Instructions: Anchor middle of a band to a secure overhead hook or bar (a bicycle hook or chin-up bar works well). You may also tie a knot in center of band and shut the knot on the other side of the top of the door. Grasp the end of the band in each hand, picking up slack so that arms are fully extended overhead. Pull your elbows toward your ribs, fully flexing your arms. Return to the start position and repeat.

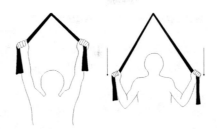

Figure 4-158

Modification (if overhead anchor is not available): Grasp the band overhead with your arms fully extended, hands about 18 inches apart. Pull your elbows to your ribs as you pull your hands apart, lowering the band in front of your face. Return to the start position and repeat.

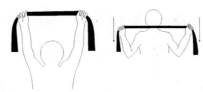

Figure 4-159. Modified: no overhead anchor

Variation: Lower your arms out to your sides without bending your elbows, so that your arms are straight and parallel to the floor, band in front of your body. Return to the start position and repeat.

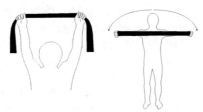

Figure 4-160. Variation: keeping elbows straight

Pullover

Purpose: Strengthens latissimus dorsi (mid-back), triceps (back of upper arm), and chest muscles, focuses on bone in spine area.

Instructions: Anchor middle of the band to a secure overhead hook or bar (a bicycle hook or chin-up bar works well). You may also tie a knot in the center of the band and shut the knot on the

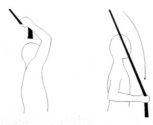

Figure 4-161

other side of the top of the door. Stand below the anchor. Grasp the end of the band in each hand, so that your arms are nearly fully extended overhead, elbows slightly flexed and the palms facing each other. Lower your arms to your sides, ending with the elbows at your ribs and bent to a 90-degree angle. Return to the start position and repeat.

Biceps Curl (With Rotation)

Purpose: Strengthens biceps (front of upper arm), focuses on bone in wrist area.

Instructions: Step on the middle of the band with one foot. Grasp ends of the band in each hand. Stand with your arms straight at your sides, *palms facing your body.* Keeping elbows "glued" to your ribs, fully flex both arms, rotating so that at full flexion, palms are facing your upper arms. Return to the start position and repeat.

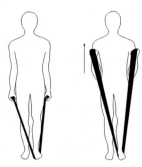

Figure 4-162

Wrist Curl/Reverse Wrist Curl

Purpose: Strengthens forearm, focuses on bone in wrist area.

Instructions:

Wrist Curl: This exercise works well using band tied in loop, though not necessary. Sit in a chair. Step on a band with one foot, grasping other end of the band in your hand. Rest your forearm on your thigh, bending from the hips and maintaining neutral lower-back curve, palm facing up with your hand extended toward the floor. Curl your hand toward the ceiling. Return to the start position and repeat.

Figure 4-163. Wrist curl

Reverse Wrist Curl: Repeat the wrist curl, only rotate the forearm so the palm faces the floor. Lift your hand toward the ceiling. Return to the start position and repeat.

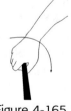

Figure 4-164. Reverse wrist curl

Wrist Rotation (pronation/supination):

Purpose: Strengthens forearm, focuses on bone in wrist area.

Instructions: This exercise works well using a band tied in a loop (though not necessary). Sit in a chair. Step on the band with one foot, grasping the other end of the band in your hand. Rest your forearm on your thigh, bending from hips and maintaining neutral lower-back curve. Rotate your wrist from side to side.

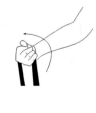

Figure 4-165

5

Stretching

Before reading this chapter, review the section on flexibility in Chapter 1. Following are brief overviews of the stretching programs that are included in this chapter. The basic programs are designed to target all joints and major muscle groups; the target programs focus more on areas of concern and can supplement a basic program.

Review of Stretching Programs

- *Basic Stretching Program: On Your Feet*—A streamlined program that includes nine stretches using all major muscle groups. You don't need any props, support, or changes in position; all exercises are done on your feet.

- *Basic Plus Stretching Program: In the Chair*—This group is a more comprehensive set of 13 exercises. This set is ideal for older adults and people in wheelchairs (depending on capability), as all exercises are performed from a chair and several include modifications. It also includes areas of the body of concern to older adults. This program does take more time; do it all when you can, and shorten when time is limited.

- *Basic Stretching Program: On the Floor*—This program is great for relaxation and taking your time with your stretching. It includes nine basic stretches, all done from the floor: sitting or lying. You must be able to easily get up and down off the floor. It is helpful to use a mat.

- *Basic Stretching Program: In Bed*—This exercise is designed for people who are ill, convalescing, or unable to get out of bed while still able to move their limbs. The 10 stretches selected are easy to perform, require a minimum of moving around, and do not require much space. In many cases, a towel or non-elastic strap will make some of the exercises easier. Modifications are pictured.

- *Target Stretches for the Back*—In general, research on back health doesn't support stretching for the spine. The stretches shown in this program—only two, both with modifications—have been shown to impose a minimum amount of stress on the spine. Please also refer to the area on strengthening for the back for a more comprehensive back care program.

- *Target Stretches for the Shoulders, and for Post-Breast or Chest Surgery*—This collection of stretches is ideal for anyone dealing with issues with the upper body: shoulder pain/injury, post-open heart surgery, post-mastectomy, post-lung surgery, and such. Start these stretches as soon as possible after surgery, moving slowly and gently, modifying range of motion as needed. Do them daily immediately post-surgery. A few weeks post-surgery, do them every other day, and intersperse with one of the other stretching programs to be sure you are including all the major muscle groups.

- Target Stretches for the Hips, Knees, and Ankles—These stretches are well suited for keeping good range of motion around the joints that keep you mobile. Maintaining or improving pliability in these joints will improve balance, walking stride, and smooth mobility, while reducing risk of pain/injury in the back, hips, knees, and ankles.

Choose a program from the previous list that best suits you and your situation (i.e., you may be unsteady and find the most security doing the seated stretches, or you may be convalescing and need to find stretches you can do while lying in bed). Conversely, you may be very active and want the most time-efficient program (On Your Feet).

Consider alternating programs and/or specific stretches. For example, as your balance improves, you may consider moving from the seated to the standing exercises (On Your Feet). Or, you may primarily perform the On Your Feet program, but prefer to add a couple stretches from the other programs when you have more time. Your body—and your mind—will welcome the variety. Mix it up.

Basic Stretching Guidelines

- Stretches may be used for cool-downs or as a part of general stretching routine done at any time.

- Hold stretch for 15 to 30 seconds. You may do one to four repetitions of each stretch. If you are just beginning and your muscles feel tight, hold just 10 seconds, and do more than one repetition. Again, vary how you do your stretches. Some days, perform more reps with a shorter holding period; other days, hold the stretch longer and perform fewer reps.

- Stretch slowly to point of mild discomfort, not pain. Do not bounce.

- Do not force painful stretching. Consult a health professional for modification or substitute exercises. Forcing stretching can aggravate an injured area.

- Muscles should be warm before stretching (therefore ideal as cool-downs after exercise). If not used as cool-downs, perform three to five minutes of light physical activity before stretching.

- Breathe normally during stretches. Do not hold your breath.

- *Pulmonary patients:* Coordinate stretches with pursed lips. Inhale before moving into stretch, exhale as you move into stretch. See Appendix E for instruction.

- *If you have a specific medical condition,* please review Specific Resistance Training Guidelines for Disabilities and Chronic Diseases A to Z (Chapter 2). Though these recommendations focus primarily on strengthening, many comments regarding stretching are included.

Basic Stretching Program: On Your Feet

This streamlined program includes nine stretches using all major muscle groups. You don't need any props, support, or changes in position. All exercises are done on your feet. Please review Basic Stretching Guidelines.

Side Stretch

Instructions: Gently stretch one arm toward the ceiling, "pushing the ceiling higher" with your palm. Lift your rib cage and shoulder blade. Maintain a neutral lower-back curve, but avoid overarching your back.

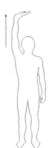

Figure 5-1

Chest Stretch

Instructions: Clasp hands behind your back while pushing both shoulders back, squeezing your shoulder blades together.

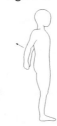

Figure 5-2

Superman Stretch

Instructions: Stand with your feet shoulder-width apart. Reach forward with both arms, focusing on spreading the shoulder blades apart. Do not lock your knees, keep your arms parallel to ground, and do not lean your torso forward.

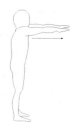

Figure 5-3

Quadriceps (Front of Thigh) Stretch

Instructions: Stand by a chair, wall, or table for support. Gently lift one heel behind you and grasp an ankle or pant leg using either hand. Stand upright and point your knee toward the floor. Repeat on other leg. If this position is difficult, support your knee on a chair seat, as pictured.

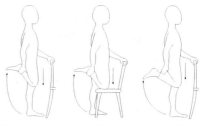

Figure 5-4. Standard, knee in chair, pant leg

Note: You can hold your foot, ankle, or pant leg with either hand: same side or opposite.

Calf Stretch

Instructions: Stand by a chair, wall, or table, using for support. Point the toes of *both* feet directly forward, bending and relaxing front leg. Gently lean your hips forward and "push" against the back heel. Repeat on the other leg (or you can stretch both legs together).

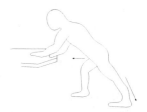

Figure 5-5

Hamstring (Back of Thigh) Stretch

Instructions: Stand with one heel on the floor in front of you. Maintaining a neutral lower-back curves, *bend from the hips* and lean your chest over the thigh. Keep your head in alignment with your spine.

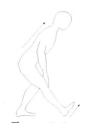

Figure 5-6

Back Scratcher

Instructions: Reach behind your head with one hand, placing it on the back of your neck with your elbow pointing toward the ceiling. Reach behind your back with the other hand so that the palm of your hand is facing out. Position the middle finger of each hand as close together as possible. Switch sides.

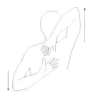

Figure 5-7

Shoulder Stretch

Instructions: Reach across your chest with one arm, laying your hand on your upper back. With your free hand, grip the elbow of the first arm and gently push your upper arm closer to your body.

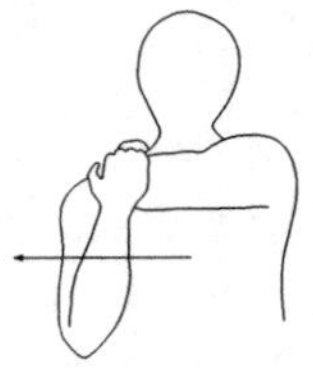

Figure 5-8

Back Twist

Instructions: Stand with good posture. Place both hands on one hip, reaching across the body with one arm. Turn your torso, shoulders, and head toward your hands, moving as a unit, looking over your shoulder. Keep your hips facing forward.

Note: Use caution when rotating your spine; do not overstretch. Be sure your muscles are warm first.

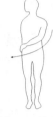

Figure 5-9

Basic *Plus* Stretching Program: In the Chair

This program is a more comprehensive set of 13 exercises. This set is ideal for older adults and people in wheelchairs (depending on capability), as all exercises are performed from a chair and several include modifications. It also includes areas of the body of concern to older adults. This program does take more time: do it all when you can and shorten when time is limited. Please review the Basic Stretching Guidelines outlined previously in this chapter.

Neck Stretches

Instructions: Sit with good posture, maintaining natural curves of the spine.

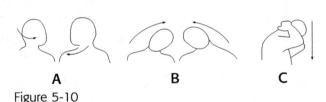

A   B   C

Figure 5-10

A: Look over one shoulder, hold; slowly roll your head across your chest, look over the other shoulder; hold.

B: Lay your ear over your shoulder, hold; repeat to the other side.

C: Lay your chin on your chest, reach behind your head, and apply gentle pressure down.

Side Stretch

Instructions: Sit with good posture, maintaining the natural curves of the spine. Gently stretch one arm toward the ceiling, pushing your palm toward the ceiling. Focus on lifting your rib cage and shoulder blade to feel the stretch through your torso.

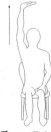

Figure 5-11

Chest Stretch

Instructions: Sit with good posture, maintaining the natural curves of the spine. Clasp your hands behind you. Push your shoulders back, squeezing your shoulder blades together. If tolerated, lift your hands higher, keeping your elbows straight.

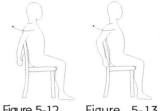

Figure 5-12   Figure 5-13. Modified

Modified: If reaching behind the chair is difficult for you, reach instead for the outside of the chair back or the arms of the chair and squeeze your shoulder blades together. If the chair has nothing to hang on to, place your hands on your hips and follow the same instructions.

Superman Stretch

Instructions: Sit with good posture, maintaining the natural curves of the spine. Reach forward in a "flying" position with both arms, pulling your shoulder blades apart and stretching through your shoulders. Alternate reaching the center, hold; "fly" to the left, hold; "fly" to the right, hold.

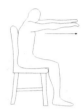

Figure 5-14

Back Scratcher

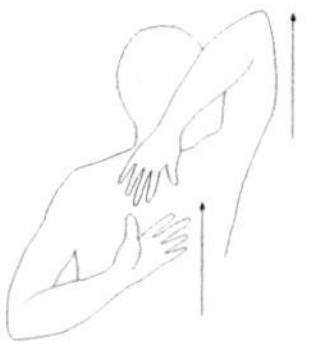

Instructions: Sit with good posture, maintaining the natural curves of the spine. Reach behind your head with one hand, placing it on back of your neck with your elbow pointing toward the ceiling. Reach behind your back with the other hand so that the palm of your hand is facing out. Position the middle finger of each hand as close together as possible. Switch.

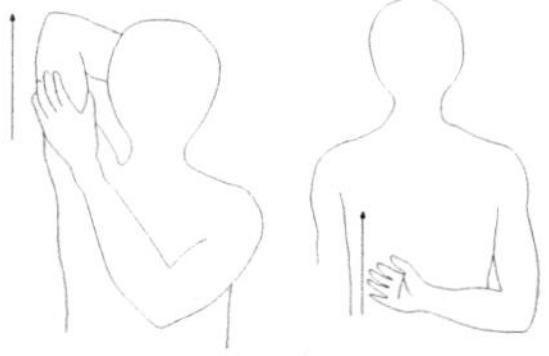

Figure 5-15

Modified: If this stretch feels uncomfortable to begin with, try doing it in two parts, just one side at a time. You may use your other hand to assist with the "elbow up" as shown in Figure 5-16.

Figure 5-16. Modified

Torso Rotation

Instructions: Sit with good posture, maintaining the natural curves of the spine. Keeping your knees pointing forward, turn your torso slowly to one side, reaching for back of chair with both hands. Look over shoulder. Hold for 15 to 30 seconds on each side.

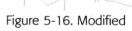
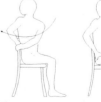

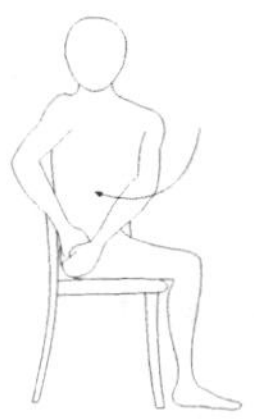

Figure 5-17   Figure 5-18. Modified

Modifed: Put both hands on the outside of your hip. Use caution against overstretching and hurting your back. Back muscles should be warm first.

Outer Hip Stretch

Instructions: Sit with good posture, maintaining the natural curves of the spine. Raise one ankle to rest on the opposite thigh, with the knee pointing out. Support your knee and ankle with both hands. While pulling your lower leg toward your chest, lean your chest over your thigh. Lead with your chin to help keep proper alignment. For variation, place your hand on top of your knee and push gently down.

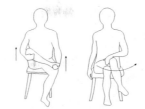

Figure 5-19   Figure 5-20

Modified: Cross one leg over the other. With the opposite hand, push the knee of the crossed leg toward your body. Do not do this exercise if you have a hip or knee replacement without specific medical release.

Ankle Rotations

Instructions: You may remain in the previous start position (see Outer Hip Stretch) or just hold foot off floor. Rotate your ankle in one direction, reverse. Follow with "point/flex." Switch. You may also "draw" half circles.

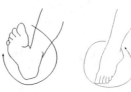

Figure 5-21

Variations:

- "Happy feet": Draw a smile (half-circle) with the foot in both directions.
- Toe point/flex: Push your toes forward, and then pull them back.

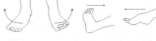

Figure 5-22. Variation: Happy feet   Figure 5-23. Variation: Toe point/flex

Inner Thigh Stretch

Instructions: Sit with your knees as wide apart as possible. Place a hand on each knee and assist in gently pushing your knees further apart.

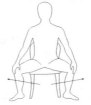

Figure 5-24

Hamstring Stretch

Instructions: Sit on the front of a chair, maintaining the natural curves of the spine Extend one leg. With your toes pointed toward the ceiling and a slight flex in the knee, lean your chest over your thigh, bending from the hip. Leading with the chin helps keep your head and spine in proper alignment. You do not need to reach the toes.

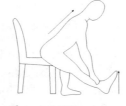

Figure 5-25

Note: Be especially careful with your posture if you have osteoporosis.

Back Stretch

Instructions: Sit with good posture, maintaining the natural curves of the spine. Lean your torso over your thighs. You may spread your knees apart and rest your elbows on your thighs if it is more comfortable. Maintain a neutral lower-back curve, and keep your head in alignment with your spine.

Figure 5-26

Note: Use caution with forward flexion with osteoporosis.

Quadriceps Stretch

Instructions: Sit toward the front of a chair with good posture, maintaining natural curves of the spine. Turn body in one direction, so that one hip is on the chair and one hip is off. Drop knee of outside leg toward floor. Keep your torso upright and push your pelvis forward. If possible, lift your heel behind you toward your hip by gripping your foot, ankle, or pant leg. Repeat on the other leg.

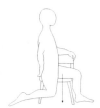

Figure 5-27

Calf Stretch

Instructions: Sit with good posture, maintaining the natural curves of the spine. Position a towel or *non*-elastic strap across the ball of one foot. Pull your toes toward your shin. You may leave your heel resting on the floor (Figure 5-28), or raise your leg parallel to the floor with your knee slightly flexed (Figure 5-29). Choose the position that feels most effective and is most comfortable to perform. Repeat on the other leg.

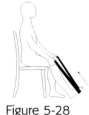

Figure 5-28   Figure   5-29.
Alternative

Basic Stretching Program: On the Floor

This program is great for relaxation and taking your time with your stretching. It includes nine basic stretches, all done from the floor: sitting or lying. You must be able to easily get up and down off the floor. It is helpful to use a mat. Please review Basic Stretching Guidelines, outlined previously in this chapter.

Inner Thigh Stretch

Instructions: Sit on floor with your heels together. If you can't get the heels together, keep your feet farther out in front of you. Sit with good posture, maintaining the natural curves of the spine. Lean your torso forward, bending from the hips. Look forward to help keep good alignment. Drop your knees toward the floor as much as comfortably possible.

Figure 5-30

Outer Thigh Stretch

Instructions: Sit cross-legged on the floor. Sit with good posture, maintaining the natural curves of the spine. Lean your torso forward, bending from the hips. Look forward to help keep good alignment. Drop your knees toward the floor as much as comfortably possible.

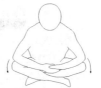

Figure 5-31

Hamstring Stretches

Choose one of the following stretches.

Instructions: Sit on floor with good posture, maintaining the natural curves of the spine. Bend one knee, bring your foot toward the inner thigh. Extend one leg out, keeping your toes pointing up to ceiling. Lean your torso slightly forward, bending from the hips. Flex your knee slightly. Keep your head in alignment with your spine.

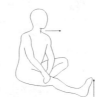

Figure 5-32

Note: Use caution with forward flexion with osteoporosis.

Variations:

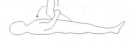

Figure 5-33

- Lie on your back and pull your thigh to your chest. Point your heel toward the ceiling, hugging your thigh to your chest.

- Lie on your back and point your heel toward the ceiling with your leg straight.

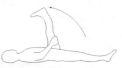

Figure 5-34

Floor Shoulder/Chest Stretch

Instructions: Sit on the floor with your knees bent. Lean back on your hands, with the angle of your hands positioned comfortably. Maintain a neutral lower-back curve. Push your shoulders back by squeezing the shoulder blades together, and slightly bend your elbows.

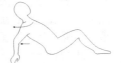

Figure 5-35

Quadriceps Stretch

Instructions: Lie on your side on the floor with both legs straight. Bend the knee of the top leg and bring your heel to your hip behind you, keeping the top thigh parallel to the floor. Do not "roll" the top hip back—keep directly over the lower hip or even slightly forward.

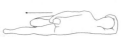

Figure 5-36

Torso Twist

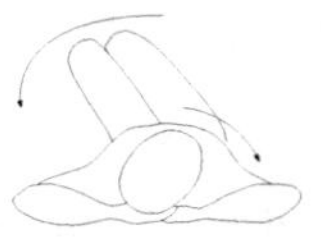

Instructions: Lie on the floor with both knees bent. Place your hands under your head or straight out to the side. Slowly lower both knees toward the floor, keeping the shoulders flat. Look in the opposite direction of the knees.

Figure 5-37

Advanced: Cross one leg over the other. Pull the crossed thigh toward the floor, keep your shoulders down, looking in the opposite direction of your knees.

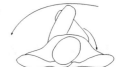

Caution: Be careful not to overtwist.

Figure 5-38. Advanced

Prone Shoulder Stretch

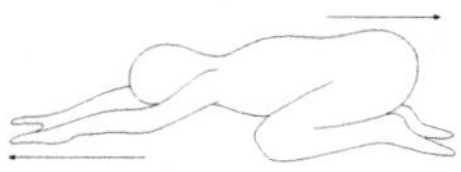

Instructions: Get on your hands and knees on the floor. Lean back until you are sitting on your calves, and reach as far forward as possible with both hands.

Figure 5-39

Full Body

Instructions: Stretch out full height with your arms overhead and toes pointed. Completely tighten all your muscles, and hold for three to five seconds. Repeat.

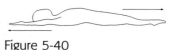

Figure 5-40

Basic Stretching Program: In Bed

These stretches are ideal for periods of illness or recovery, when getting out of bed is difficult. Gentle stretching during these times will help to reduce loss in range of motion and deconditioning that rapidly occurs with bed rest, as well as just feeling better in general. For best results, combine with Basic Resistance Training Program: In Bed (Chapter 4).

As with all stretches, it is helpful to warm the muscles first. A modified "walking in place"—bending the knees and moving the arms—can be performed in a horizontal position in most circumstances. Any kind of light intensity, rhythmical movement, such as modified leg raises (one at a time) or heel lifts, will work fine. All activity and stretches described in the following exercises should be well within your capability. Please review Basic Stretching Guidelines, outlined previously in this chapter.

Light Physical Activity/Warm-Up

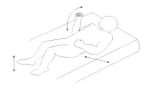

Instructions: Depending on your ability to safely move, find a way to do a few minutes of light physical activity, perhaps a modified walking in place, using your arms if possible.

Figure 5-41

Hamstring Stretch

Instructions: Lie on your back. Pull your knee to your chest. Grasp your thigh, knee, or calf with both hands. Straighten your leg as much as possible (though maintaining a slight flex), pointing your heel to the ceiling and pointing your toes down toward you.

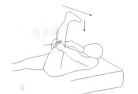

Figure 5-42

Modified: Use a towel or non-elastic strap to help support your leg. Repeat on the other leg. Point your heel toward the ceiling and point your toes down toward you.

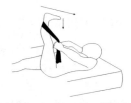

Figure 5-43. Modified: Use towel or non-elastic strap

Calf Stretch

Instructions: Lie on your back. Pull your knee to your chest. Position a towel or non-elastic strap across the ball of your foot. Extend your leg toward the ceiling and pull your toes toward you using a towel or strap. Repeat on the other leg.

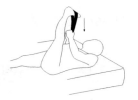

Figure 5-44. Use towel or non-elastic strap

Hip Abduction

Instructions: Lie on your back. Pull your knee to your chest. Place one hand on your knee and one on your foot. Pull your foot toward your body with knee your pointing out. Pull both your knee and your foot up toward body.

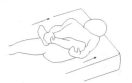

Figure 5-45

Modified: Position a towel or non-elastic strap across middle of your foot. Use a strap or towel to assist in the previous directions.

Note: Do not do this exercise if you have had a hip or knee replacement without permission from your physician.

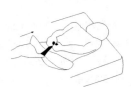

Figure 5-46. Modified: Use towel or non-elastic strap

Quadriceps Stretch

Instructions: Lie on your side. Bend the knee of your top leg, bringing your heel behind you. Keep your knee pointing straight down toward the other foot. Grasp the ankle or foot of the bent leg. Do not roll your hip backward nor bend at the hip—keep the top hip directly over the bottom hip.

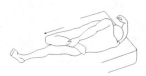

Figure 5-47

Modified: Position a towel or non-elastic strap across your ankle or the middle of your foot. Use a strap or towel to assist in the previous directions.

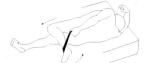

Figure 5-48. Modified: Use towel or non-elastic strap

Shoulder Stretch

Instructions: Lie on your back. Bring one arm across your body. Either keep your elbow only slightly flexed and allow your hand to rest on the bed on the other side, or bend your elbow and tuck your hand/forearm behind your head/neck (whichever is more comfortable). With your other hand, push the elbow of your first arm closer to your body.

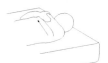

Figure 5-49

Chest Stretch

Instructions: Lie on your back. Clasp your hands behind your head. Push your elbows into the bed on both sides.

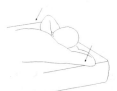

Figure 5-50

Ceiling Stretch

Instructions: Lie on your back. Reach both arms toward the ceiling, with your elbows straight and your palms facing each other. Lift both shoulders off the bed as you reach.

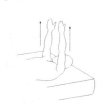

Figure 5-51

Overhead Stretch

Instructions: Lie on your back. Place your hands behind your head, and reach down your neck/upper back as much as possible. Push your elbows straight overhead. Try to stretch through your torso, lifting your ribs and shoulder blades.

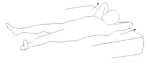

Figure 5-52

Torso Stretch

Instructions: Lie on your back. Bend both knees. Place your hands under your head or out to the side. Slowly and gently roll the knees in one direction, keeping your shoulders flat against bed and look in the opposite direction of your knees. Be careful not to overtwist.

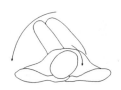

Figure 5-53

Target Stretches for the Back

According to back expert Stuart McGill (2001), most back flexibility exercises (such as the popular "knee to chest") do not improve back health nor lessen risk of injury, contrary to popular belief. In fact, greater spinal mobility is not necessarily helpful when the back is injured. Most of the following guidelines also come from his extensive research. Follow these guidelines for stretching related to back health (for strengthening guidelines regarding back health, see Chapter 4):

- Greater flexibility at the hips and knees seems to provide benefit. See the stretches in this section.
- Always maintain the natural curves of the spine. A "neutral lower-back curve" is the most stable position.
- The popular "pelvic tilt," often used in back exercises, is not recommended, as no evidence suggests that it prevents injury during lifting or exertion, and it actually increases load on the spine.
- Spine flexibility should not be emphasized when the back is injured until the spine is "stabilized" and has been conditioned with strength and endurance exercise.
- Avoid full-range back stretches (such as "knee/knees to chest") first thing in the morning.
- Aerobic exercise, such as walking, is one of the best activities to both treat as well as reduce the risk of lower-back injury, especially first-time back injury.
- Perform back exercises every day (see Chapter 4 for strengthening exercises).
- Have patience and be compliant. Reduced pain and better function may not occur for up to three months.

The following flexibility exercises have been selected for minimizing load on the spine and are based on knowledge of how back injuries occur. More fit people can tolerate more loading. These stretches are best suited for the person beginning a post-injury program or someone at risk for injuring their back.

Slow Lunges

Instructions: Stand with one foot in front of the other. Keep your torso upright at all times, maintaining a neutral lower-back curve. Slowly lunge forward, bending the front knee at no greater than a 90-degree angle. Switch. Perform 10 to 15 lunges on each leg.

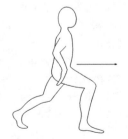

Figure 5-54

Hip Flexion (Hamstring Stretch)

Instructions: Stand as pictured in Figure 5-55 with your foot resting on an object that raises leg up to a 90-degree angle. Maintain a neutral lower-back curve. Extend one leg in front of you. Flex the knee slightly. Hold for 15 to 30 seconds.

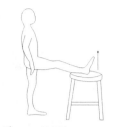

Figure 5-55

Variations:

- Perform from a chair if necessary.
- On the floor instead of standing, lie on the floor and rest your heels on the wall. Keep your feet flexed as much as possible. Try to rest in this position, holding as long as two to three minutes if possible. Work on positioning your hips closer to the wall as flexibility improves.

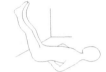

Figure 5-56. Variation

Cat Stretch

Instructions: Get on your hands and knees. Slowly cycle from full spine flexion to full extension. Repeat 10 to 15 times in both directions.

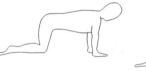
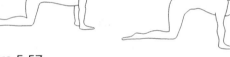

Figure 5-57

Variation: This exercise can also be done from a seated position.

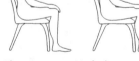

Figure 5-58. Variation

Target Stretches for the Shoulders and for Post-Breast or Chest Surgery

This collection of stretches is ideal for anyone dealing with issues with the upper body: shoulder pain/injury, post-open heart surgery, post-mastectomy, post-lung surgery, and the like. Start these stretches as soon as possible after surgery, moving slowly and gently. Do them daily immediately post-surgery. A few weeks post-surgery, do them every other day, and intersperse with one of the other stretching programs to be sure you are including all the major muscle groups. Please review Basic Stretching Guidelines, outlined previously in this chapter.

Pendulum Exercise

Purpose: Increases range of motion in all directions of shoulder joints; relaxes and loosens shoulder joints.

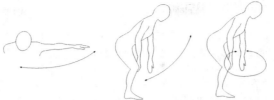

Part 1 **Part 2** **Part 3**

Figure 5-59

Instructions: Bend forward so that your torso is between a 45-degree angle and parallel to floor. Support the torso by resting your arm on a table, chair back, counter, or your thigh. Note: Do not rest your full body weight on your affected arm. Maintain a neutral lower-back curve and tighten abdominals to protect your back. Perform Parts 1 to 3; switch arms.

- Part 1: Slowly sweep your arm from side to side (left to right). Do 8 to 12 repetitions.

- Part 2: Slowly sweep your arm forward and backward (head to leg). Do 8 to 12 repetitions.

- Part 3: Slowly rotate your arm in a wide circle; first in one direction, then in the other. Do 8 to 12 repetitions each way.

Head Hug

Purpose: Increases range of motion in shoulder, underarm, chest.

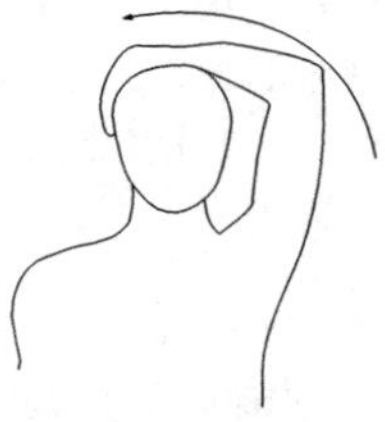

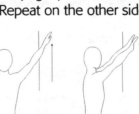

Figure 5-60

Instructions: Place the fingertips of the affected arm over the ear, with your elbow pointing out to the side. "Walk" the finger over the top of the head to the other ear, keeping your elbow pointing out to the side. Keep your head in an upright position. Return your fingertips to the other ear. Do 8 to 12 repetitions. Repeat on the other side.

Wall Walk

Purpose: Increases the range of motion in shoulder abduction.

Instructions:

Part 1 **Part 2**

Figure 5-61

- Part 1: Stand with your side to the wall. "Walk" your fingers up the wall as high as possible. Return to start, trying to reach a little higher each time. Do 8 to 12 repetitions. Switch sides.

- Part 2: Stand facing the wall. "Walk" the fingers of both arms up the wall as high as possible. Return to the start, trying to reach a little higher each time. Do 8 to 12 repetitions.

Note: For both exercises, step closer to wall as range of motion improves

Back Scratcher

Purpose: Improves the range of motion of internal and external rotators of shoulders.

Instructions: Slowly reach behind your head with one hand, placing it on the back of your head or neck (depending on range of motion) with your elbow pointing toward the ceiling. Reach behind your back with the other hand so that the palm of your hand is facing out. Work on decreasing the distance between the middle finger of each hand. Hold for 15 to 30 seconds. Switch sides.

Modified: You can split exercise into two parts.

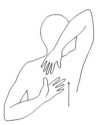

Figure 5-62

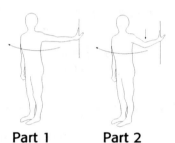

Figure 5-63. Modified

Chest Stretch

Purpose: Stretches chest, shoulder, and upper arm muscles; stretches skin across incision and chest wall.

Instructions: Place your hand about shoulder height on a wall or doorframe with your fingers pointing back and your thumb up toward the ceiling.

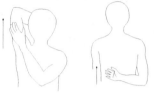

Part 1　　　**Part 2**

Figure 5-64

- Part 1: For upper arm: With your elbow straight, slowly turn your feet and torso away from your hand. Hold for five seconds. Do 8 to 12 repetitions. Switch sides.
- Part 2: For chest: With your elbow bent, slowly turn your feet and torso away from your hand. Hold for five seconds. Do 8 to 12 repetitions. Switch sides.

Superman Stretch

Purpose: Stretches upper back muscles.

Instructions: Reach forward in a "flying" position with both arms, pulling your shoulder blades apart and stretching through the shoulders. Alternate reaching center, hold; "fly" to left, hold; "fly" right, hold. Hold each side for 15 to 30 seconds.

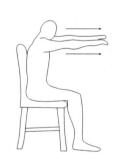

Figure 5-65

Clasped Overhead Hold

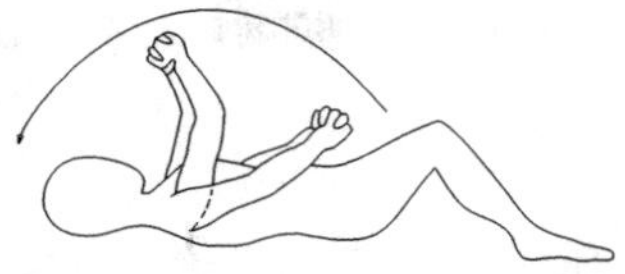

Purpose: Improves the range of motion of shoulders and underarm.

Figure 5-66

Instructions: Lie on the bed or floor with your knees bent and your feet flat. Clasp your hands and lift your arms overhead, keeping your elbows slightly flexed. Stop when you feel tightness; relax your arms. Hold for one minute, gradually increasing to 10 minutes.

Note: If you are just starting, you may want to put one or two pillows above your head to rest arms on.

Wide Arc Overhead Hold

Purpose: Improves the range of motion of shoulder abductors and chest muscles.

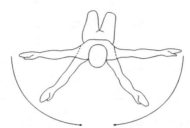

Instructions: Lie on the bed or floor with your knees bent and your feet flat. Position your arms straight by your side. Keeping your arms straight, your elbows and wrists on the floor, and your palms up (if possible), move your arms out to the side and as high as possible. Hold for one minute, gradually increasing to 10 minutes with your arms all the way up.

Figure 5-67

Elbow Hold

Purpose: Improves the range of motion of shoulder and chest muscles.

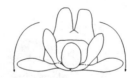

Figure 5-68

Instructions: Lie on the bed or floor with your knees bent and feet flat. Position your hands behind your head with your elbows pointing toward the ceiling. Let your elbows drop gently toward the floor. Hold in a dropped position for one minute, gradually increasing to 10 minutes.

Note: If you are just starting, you may want to put pillows under your elbows.

Full Body Stretch

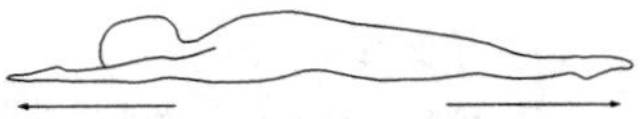

Purpose: Stretches and relaxes the entire body.

Figure 5-69

Instructions: Lie on the bed or floor with your arms overhead and as straight as is comfortable. Stretch your body from end to end as far as possible with a long exhalation. Relax the entire body, keeping your arms overhead. Concentrate on slow, deep breaths. Repeat two to three times. Relax in this position for several minutes, if possible.

Target Stretches for the Hips, Knees, and Ankles

These stretches are well suited for keeping a good range of motion around the joints that keep you mobile. Maintaining or improving pliability in these joints will improve balance, walking stride, and smooth mobility, while reducing risk of pain/injury in the back, hips, knees, and ankles. Use caution if you have had a knee or hip replacement. Consult your physician if you have questions regarding any of these stretches. Please review Basic Stretching Guidelines, outlined previously in this chapter.

Quadriceps Stretches

Purpose: Stretches front of thigh.

Choose one of the following stretches.

❏ Standing

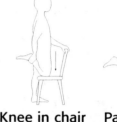

Standard   Knee in chair   Pant leg

Figure 5-70

Instructions: Stand by a chair, wall, or table for support. Gently lift one heel behind you and grasp your ankle or pant leg, using either hand. Stand upright and point your knee toward the floor. Repeat on the other leg. If this position is difficult, support your knee on chair seat, as pictured in Figure 5-70.

Note: You can hold foot, ankle, or pant leg with either hand: same side or opposite.

❏ In chair

Instructions: Sit toward the front of the chair with good posture, maintaining the natural curves of the spine. Turn your body in one direction, so that one hip is on the chair and one hip is off. Drop the knee of your outside leg toward the floor. Keep your torso upright, and push your pelvis forward. If possible, lift the heel behind you toward your hip by gripping your foot, ankle, or pant leg. Repeat on the other leg.

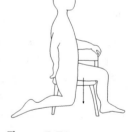

Figure 5-71

❏ On floor

Instructions: Lie on your side on the floor with both legs straight. Bend the knee of your top leg and bring your heel to the hip behind you, keeping the top thigh parallel to the floor. Do not "roll" the top hip back—keep directly over the lower hip or even slightly forward.

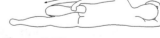

Figure 5-72

❏In bed

Instructions: Lie on your side. Bend the knee of your top leg, bringing your heel behind you. Keep your knee pointing straight down toward the other foot. Grasp the ankle or foot of your bent leg. Do not roll your hip backward nor bend at your hip; keep your top hip directly over your bottom hip.

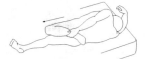

Figure 5-73

Modified: Position a towel or non-elastic strap across your ankle or the middle of your foot. Use the strap or towel to assist in the previous directions.

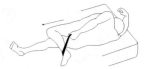

Figure 5-74. Modified: Use towel or non-elastic strap

Hamstring Stretches

Purpose: Stretches back of the thigh.

Choose one of the following stretches.

❏Standing

Instructions: Stand with one heel on the floor in front of you. Maintaining a neutral lower-back curve, bend from the hips and lean your chest over your thigh. Keep your head in alignment with your spine.

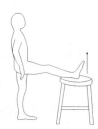

Figure 5-75

❏In chair

Instructions: Sit on the front of the chair, maintaining the natural curves of the spine Extend one leg. With your toes pointed toward the ceiling and a slight flex in the knee, lean your chest over your thigh, bending from the hip. Leading with the chin helps keep your head and spine in proper alignment. You do not need to reach the toes

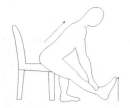

Figure 5-76

Note: Be especially careful with your posture if you have osteoporosis.

❏On floor

Instructions: Sit on the floor with good posture, maintaining the natural curves of the spine. Extend one leg out, keeping your toes pointing up to the ceiling. Lean your torso forward, bending from the hips. Flex your knee slightly. Keep your head in alignment with your spine.

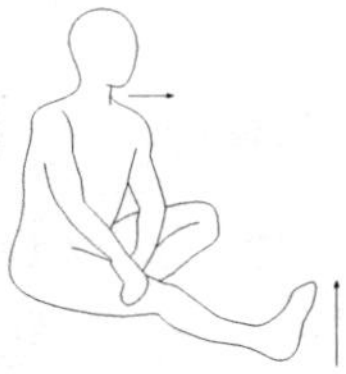

Figure 5-77

Variations:

- Lie on your back and pull your thigh to your chest. Point your heel toward the ceiling, hugging your thigh to your chest.

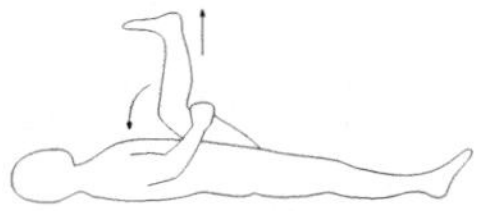

Figure 5-78. Variation

- Lie on your back and point your heel toward the ceiling with your leg straight.

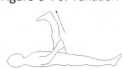

Figure 5-79. Variation

❏In bed

Instructions: Lie on your back. Pull your knee to your chest. Grasp your thigh, knee, or calf with both hands. Straighten your leg as much as possible (though maintaining a slight flex), pointing your heel to the ceiling and pointing your toes down toward you.

Modified: Use a towel or non-elastic strap to help support your leg. Repeat on the other leg.

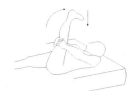

Figure 5-80

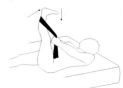

Figure 5-81. Modified: Use towel or non-elastic strap

Inner Thigh Stretches

Purpose: Stretches inner thigh.

Choose one of the following stretches.

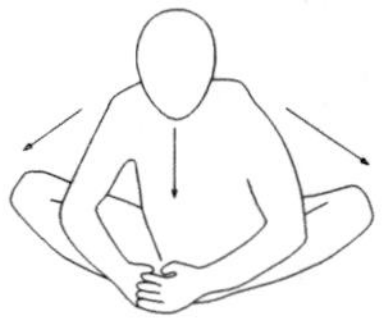

❏On floor

Instructions: Sit on the floor with your heels together. If you can't get the heels together, keep your feet farther out in front of you. Sit with good posture, maintaining the natural curves of the spine. Lean your torso forward, bending from the hips. Look forward to help keep good alignment. Drop your knees toward the floor as much as comfortably possible.

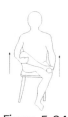

Figure 5-82

❏In chair

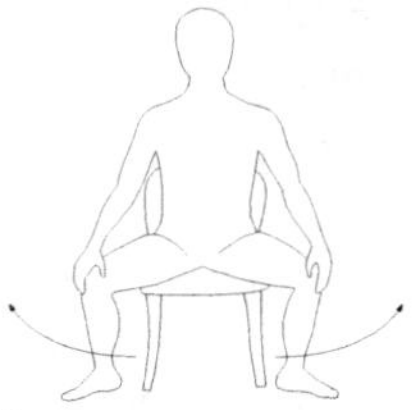

Instructions: Sit with your knees as wide apart as possible. Place a hand on each knee, and assist in gently pushing the knees further apart.

Figure 5-83

Outer Thigh Stretches

Note: Do not do these stretches if you have a hip or knee replacement without specific medical release.

Purpose: Stretches outer thigh.

Choose one of the following stretches.

❏In chair

Instructions: Sit with good posture, maintaining the natural curves of the spine. Raise one ankle to rest on the opposite thigh, with your knee pointing out. Support your knee and ankle with both

Figure 5-84

hands. While pulling your lower leg toward your chest, lean your chest over your thigh. Lead with the chin to help keep proper alignment. For variation, place your hand on top of your knee and push gently down.

Modified: Cross one leg over the other. With the opposite hand, push the knee of your crossed leg toward your body.

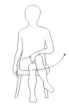

Figure 5-85. Modified

❑On floor

Instructions: Sit cross-legged on the floor. Sit with good posture, maintaining the natural curves of the spine. Lean your torso forward, bending from the hips. Look forward to help keep good alignment. Drop your knees toward the floor as much as comfortably possible.

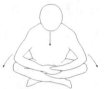

Figure 5-86

❑On floor or in bed

Instructions: Lie on your back on the floor or in bed. Bend one knee. Position the ankle of other leg on the thigh near the knee of first leg, with the knee of the second leg pointing out to the side. Grasp the thigh of the first leg with both hands. Pull the thigh gently toward your chest.

Figure 5-87

Calf Stretches

Purpose: Stretches calf.

Choose one of the following stretches.

❑Standing

Instructions: Stand by a chair, wall, or table, using for support. Point the toes of both feet directly forward, bending and relaxing the front leg. Gently lean the hips forward and push against your back heel. Repeat on the other leg (or you can stretch both legs together).

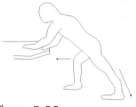

Figure 5-88

❑In chair

Instructions: Sit with good posture, maintaining the natural curves of the spine. Position a towel or non-elastic strap across ball of one foot. Pull your toes toward your shin. You may leave your heel resting on the floor (Figure 5-89), or raise your leg parallel to the floor with the knee slightly flexed (Figure 5-90). Choose the position that feels most effective and is most comfortable to perform. Repeat on the other leg.

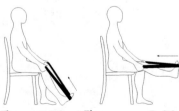

Figure 5-89   Figure   5-90. Alternative

❑On floor or in bed

Instructions: Lie on your back. Pull your knee to your chest. Position a towel or non-elastic strap across the ball of your foot. Extend your leg toward the ceiling and pull your toes toward you using the towel or strap. Repeat on the other leg.

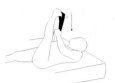

Figure 5-91. Modified: Use towel or non-elastic strap

Hip Flexor Stretch

Purpose: Stretches front upper thigh.

Instructions: Rest on one knee and one foot. Both legs should be bent to a 90-degree angle. Lean forward until the stretch is felt in the front upper thigh. Keep the front knee over your toes and your torso upright.

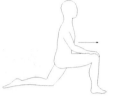

Figure 5-92

Ankle Rotations/Flexion

Purpose: Improves the range of motion of the ankle joint and lower limb muscles and tendons.

Instructions: Lift your foot off the floor. Rotate your ankle in one direction, reverse. Follow with "point/flex." Switch. You may also "draw" half circles (happy feet).

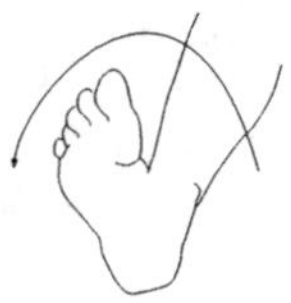

Figure 5-93

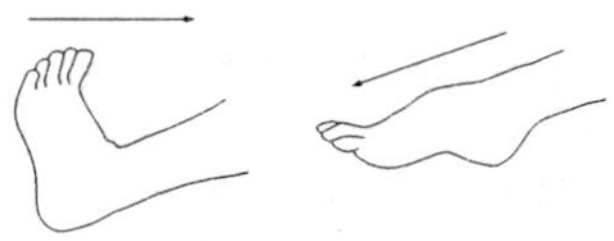

Figure 5-94. Point/flex

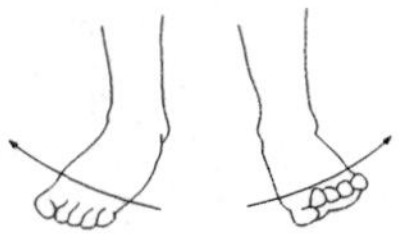

Figure 5-95. Happy feet

6

Balancing

Basic Balance Guidelines

- Always stand with good posture (see Chapter 3).
- Relax muscles and establish slow, deep breathing.
- Stand tall with lifted rib cage.
- Keep eyes looking forward, focused on a visual target at about eye level.
- Do not try more challenging balance activities until you have mastered the less challenging activities. For example, don't try closing your eyes if you are unsteady with eyes open. Don't stand on softer or unstable surfaces, such as foam and stability rocker boards, until you can balance on a hard surface.
- If you are unsteady, do these activities with your back to a wall at a distance of about two feet, and have a chair in front of you.
- If you are practicing a balance activity with your eyes closed and you feel you may lose your balance, open your eyes immediately.
- When using unstable surfaces, practice getting safely on and off, transferring weight slowly. Practice getting on and off in a forward, backward, and side position.

Beginning Balance Program

Standing With Good Posture

Instructions:

- Begin by establishing good posture (see Chapter 3).

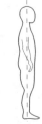

Figure 6-1

Standing With Feet Together

Instructions:

- Stand with good posture with your feet together—hold for 5 to 15 seconds.
- Stand with your feet together and your eyes closed—hold for 5 to 15 seconds.
- Stand with your feet together and arms crossed over your chest—hold for 5 to 15 seconds.
- Stand with your feet together, arms across your chest, and your eyes closed—hold for 5 to 15 seconds.

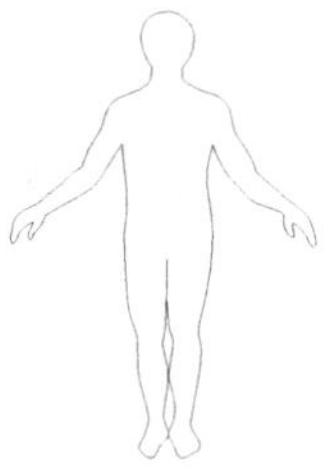

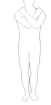

Figure 6-2.
Feet together

Figure 6-3.
Feet together, arms crossed over chest

Semi-Tandem Position

Instructions:

- Stand in a semi-tandem position (one foot behind your front foot, with a small space between the feet)—hold for 5 to 15 seconds.
- Stand in a semi-tandem position with your eyes closed—hold for 5 to 15 seconds.
- Stand in a semi-tandem position with arms across your chest—hold for 5 to 15 seconds.
- Stand in a semi-tandem position with arms across your chest and your eyes closed—hold for 5 to 15 seconds.

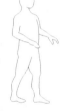

Figure 6-4.
Semi-tandem position

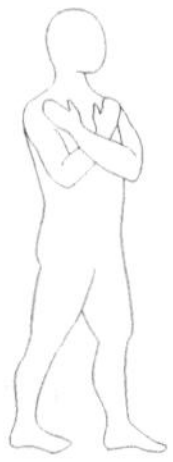

Figure 6-5.
Semi-tandem position, with arms across chest

Tandem Position

Instructions:

- Stand in a tandem position (one foot directly behind the other, toe of front foot against heel of front foot).
- Stand in a tandem position with your eyes closed—hold for 5 to 15 seconds.
- Stand in a tandem position with arms across your chest—hold for 5 to15 seconds.
- Stand in a tandem position with arms across your chest and your eyes closed—hold for 5 to 15 seconds.

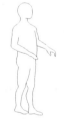
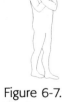

Figure 6-6.
Tandem position

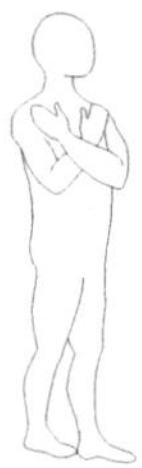

Figure 6-7.
Tandem position, with arms across chest

Standing on One Foot (Modified)

Instructions:

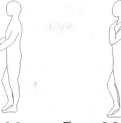

- Stand with one foot off the ground. You may rest toe lightly on the floor, on top of your other foot, or on your opposite leg—hold for 5 to 15 seconds.

Figure 6-8.
One foot
(modified)

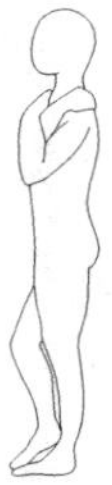

Figure 6-9.
One foot
(modified),
with arms
across chest

- Stand with one foot off the ground with your eyes closed—hold for 5 to 15 seconds.

- Stand with one foot off the ground with arms across your chest—hold for 5 to 15 seconds.

- Stand with one foot off the ground with arms across your chest and your eyes closed—hold for 5 to 15 seconds.

Intermediate Balance Program

Heel Lift

Instructions:

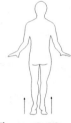

- Stand with your feet shoulder-width apart.
- Extend your arms slightly forward, lower than your shoulders.
- Lift both heels off the floor—hold for 10 to 30 seconds.

Figure 6-10

Foot to Ankle

Instructions:

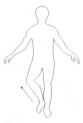

- Stand with your feet shoulder-width apart.
- Place one foot on the inside of the opposite ankle with your knee pointing out to the side—hold for 10 to 30 seconds.
- Repeat with the other foot.

Figure 6-11

One-Legged Stand—Forward

Instructions:

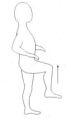

- Stand with your feet shoulder-width apart.
- Lift one knee in front of you to hip level; switch—hold for 10 to 30 seconds
- Repeat with the other leg.

Figure 6-12

One-Legged Stand—Backward

Instructions:

- Stand with your feet shoulder-width apart.
- Lift one heel behind you to knee level; switch—hold for 10 to 30 seconds
- Repeat with the other leg.

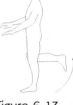

Figure 6-13

Leg Raise Front-to-Back

Instructions:

- Stand with your feet shoulder-width apart.
- Raise your leg in front of your body, moving from the hip.
- Move your leg behind your body, keeping your foot off the floor and moving from the hip

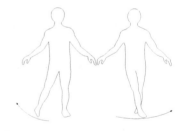

Figure 6-14

- Perform these movements for 10 to 30 seconds, then repeat with the other leg.

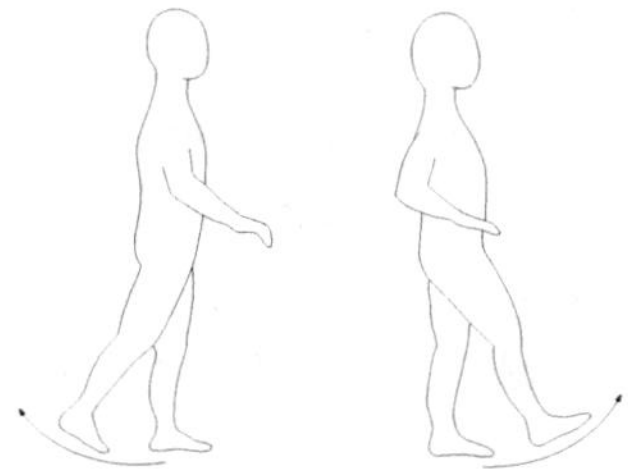

Leg Raise Side-to-Side

Instructions:

- Stand with your feet shoulder-width apart.
- Raise your leg out to the side of your body, moving from the hip, and then cross in front of the other leg.
- Raise your leg out to the side of your body, then cross behind the other leg; switch.
- Perform these movements for 10 to 30 seconds, then repeat with the other leg.

Figure 6-15

APPENDIX: "HERE TO HELP" TOOLS AND REFERENCES

©2009 Jupiter Images Corporation

Appendix

Appendix A
The Fitness Tripod: Detailed Version

Fitness is primarily comprised of three components, and can be thought of as a three-legged tripod. If all legs are not well in place, the tripod is wobbly and at risk of falling. The three legs of fitness are identified and described in the following diagram. For discussion, see Chapter 1

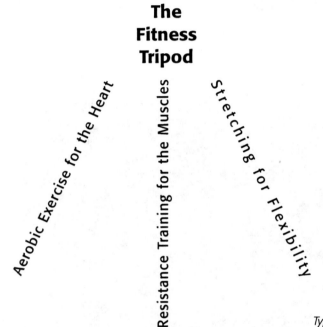

The Fitness Tripod

Aerobic Exercise for the Heart

Resistance Training for the Muscles

Stretching for Flexibility

Cardiovascular Endurance

Type of exercise: Aerobic ("with oxygen")

Frequency: 3, preferably 5x/week

Intensity: Moderate (RPE 11-13) to vigorous (RPE 13-15).

Duration: 20-50 minutes, intermittent or continuous

Examples: Walking, cycling, swimming, rowing, hiking

Benefits: Increased heart-lung fitness, exercise tolerance, energy, improved blood lipids blood sugar tolerance, and body composition. Decreased blood pressure and heart rate.

Muscular Strength/Endurance

Type of exercise: Resistance training

Frequency: 2-3x/week

Intensity: Moderate (RPE 12-13), increasing to hard (RPE 15) after 8-12 weeks, if stable and no symptoms.

Repetitions: 1 set of 8-15 initially, increasing to 2-3 sets if tolerated and if desired

Examples: Hand weights, elastic bands, resistance machines (e.g., Nautilus)

Benefits: Increased muscle mass, strength, endurance, energy, balance, coordination, walking speed/distance, bone density, metabolism, blood sugar control. Decreased load on heart, blood pressure, risk of injury, back pain, body fat, risk of frailty, and loss of independence. with "resistance training"

Flexibility

Type of exercise: Stretching exercises

Frequency: 3-7x/week

Intensity: Mild discomfort

Duration: 15-30 seconds each

Examples: Cool-down stretches

Benefits: Increased range of motion of joints, mobility, coordination, joint stability. Decreased stiffness, joint pain, risk of injury.

Appendix B
PAR-Q and You: "Readiness to Exercise" Questionnaire

The Physical Activity Readiness Questionnaire — PAR-Q *(revised 2002)*
PAR-Q & YOU (A Questionnaire for People Aged 15 to 69)

Regular physical activity is fun and healthy, and increasingly more people are starting to become more active every day. Being more active is very safe for most people. However, some people should check with their doctor before they start becoming much more physically active.

If you are planning to become much more physically active than you are now, start by answering the seven questions below. If you are between the ages of 15 and 69, the PAR-Q will tell you if you should check with your doctor before you start. If you are over 69 years of age, and you are not used to being very active, check with your doctor.

Common sense is your best guide when you answer these questions. Please read the questions carefully and answer each one honestly: check YES or NO.

YES	NO	
☐	☐	1. Has your doctor ever said that you have a heart condition and that you should only do physical activity recommended by a doctor?
☐	☐	2. Do you feel pain in your chest when you do physical activity?
☐	☐	3. In the past month, have you had chest pain when you were not doing physical activity?
☐	☐	4. Do you lose your balance because of dizziness or do you ever lose consciousness?
☐	☐	5. Do you have a bone or joint problem (for example, back, knee, or hip) that could be made worse by a change in your physical activity?
☐	☐	6. Is your doctor currently prescribing drugs (for example, water pills) for your blood pressure or heart condition?
☐	☐	7. Do you know of any other reason why you should not do physical activity?

If you answered

YES to one or more questions:

Talk with your doctor by phone or in person BEFORE you start becoming much more physically active or BEFORE you have a fitness appraisal. Tell your doctor about the PAR-Q and which questions you answered YES.
- You may be able to do any activity you want—as long as you start slowly and build up gradually. Or, you may need to restrict your activities to those that are safe for you. Talk with your doctor about the kinds of activities you wish to participate in and follow his/her advice.
- Find out which community programs are safe and helpful for you.

NO to all questions

If you answered NO honestly to all PAR-Q questions, you can be reasonably sure that you can:
- Start becoming much more physically active—begin slowly and build up gradually. This is the safest and easiest way to go.
- Take part in a fitness appraisal—this is an excellent way to determine your basic fitness so that you can plan the best way for you to live actively. It is also highly recommended that you have your blood pressure evaluated. If your reading is over 144/94, talk with your doctor before you start becoming much more physically active.

DELAY BECOMING MUCH MORE ACTIVE:
- If you are not feeling well because of a temporary illness such as a cold or a fever—wait until you feel better; or
- If you are or may be pregnant—talk to your doctor before you start becoming more active.

PLEASE NOTE: If your health changes so that you then answer YES to any of the above questions, tell your fitness or health professional. Ask whether you should change your physical activity plan.

<u>Informed Use of the PAR-Q:</u> The Canadian Society for Exercise Physiology, Health Canada, and their agents assume no liability for persons who undertake physical activity, and if in doubt after completing this questionnaire, consult your doctor prior to physical activity.

No changes permitted. You are encouraged to copy the PAR-Q but only if you use the entire form.

Note: If the PAR-Q is being given to a person before he or she participates in a physical activity program or a fitness appraisal, this section may be used for legal or administrative purposes.

I have read, understood, and completed this questionnaire. Any questions I had were answered to my full satisfaction.

NAME _____

SIGNATURE _____   DATE _____

SIGNATURE OF PARENT _____   WITNESS _____
OR GUARDIAN (FOR PARTICIPANTS UNDER THE AGE OF MAJORITY)

> **Note: This physical activity clearance is valid for a maximum of 12 months from the date it is completed and becomes invalid if your condition changes so that you would answer YES to any of the seven questions.**

© Canadian Society for Exercise Physiology
Societe canadienne de physiologie de l'exercice

Supported by: Health   Santé
Canada   Canada

Source: The Physical Activity Readiness Questionnaire — PAR-Q (revised 2002). Reprinted with permission from the Canadian Society for Exercise Physiology. www.csep.ca/forms.asp

Appendix C
Monitoring Exercise Intensity With Heart Rate

To determine your estimated target heart rate (HR), use one of the following methods.

Resting Heart Rate (RHR) + 20 to 40:

Some medications alter heart rate, making the given formulas inappropriate. Ask your physician if you are taking anything that affects heart rate. If so, this simple formula is often effective:

Resting heart rate + 20 to 40 beats per minute

In other words, try to get the heart rate at least 20 beats/minute over resting level, but not over 40 beats/minute. This method can also be safe and effective for people just beginning a program.

Percent of HRmax

The best way to obtain your maximum heart rate is by a maximal stress test administered by your physician. In the absence of this true HRmax, you can predict your HRmax by this equation (use only if you know you are not on medications that alter heart rate):

- Step 1: 220 minus age = HRmax
- Step 2: Multiply HRmax by 70 to 85 percent to obtain target HR range (may start lower) (70 to 85 percent approximates 55 to 75 percent of maximal oxygen uptake)
  - ✓ (220 - age) x .70 = lower end of range
  - ✓ (220 - age) x .85 = upper end of range

Example

- 220 - 60 = 160 (Estimated HRmax)
- 160 x .70 = 112 (70 percent HRmax: lower end of target HR)
- 106 x .85 = 136 (85 percent HRmax: upper end of target HR)
- Target heart rate for 60-year-old: 112 to 136

Heart Rate Reserve

This formula also estimates your HRmax as described in the previous section, but also incorporates your resting heart rate (use only if you know you are not on medications that alter HR).

- Step 1: 220 - age = Max HR
- Step 2: Subtract Resting HR from Max HR
- Step 3: Multiply that number by 60 to 80 percent to obtain target HR range (may start lower) (60 to 80 percent approximates 60 to 80 percent maximal oxygen uptake

- Step 4: Add Resting HR to number
  - ✓ (220 - age) - Rest HR x .60 + Rest HR = lower end of range
  - ✓ (220 - age) - Rest HR x .80 + Rest HR = upper end of range

Example

- 220 - 60 = 160 (Estimated HRmax)
- (160 - 70) = 90 x .60 = 54 + 70 = 124 (60 percent: low end of target HR)
- (160 - 70) = 90 x .80 = 72 + 70 = 142 (60 percent: low end of target HR)
- Target heart rate for 60-year-old: 124 to 142

To determine your heart rate while exercising, count your pulse for 10 seconds, and multiply the number by six. To locate your pulse:

- Drop your first two or three fingers (not your thumb) over the hollow that rests below the bone that comes off the thumb at the underside of the wrist.
- Lay your fingers over your Adam's apple and slide over hollow alongside the Adam's apple. Be sure not to press too hard.

Appendix D
Reference Scales

Rating of Perceived Exertion (RPE) Scale

6	
7	Very, very light
8	
9	Very light
10	
11	Fairly light
12	
13	Somewhat hard
14	
15	Hard
16	
17	Very hard
18	
19	Very, very hard
20	

Source: Borg, GAV. *Med Sci. Sports Exerc.*, 14: 377-381, 1982.

Breathlessness Scale

0	Not at all
0.5	Just noticeable
1	Very slight
2	Slight
3	Moderate
4	Somewhat severe
5	Severe
6	
7	Very severe
8	
9	
10	Very, very severe

Keep level of breathlessness at 4 or less.

Rating of Pain Scale

0	No pain at all
1	
2	Fairly low
3	
4	
5	Moderate
6	
7	
8	Significant
9	
10	The worst pain you can imagine

This scale is to help you define your pain level. It can be used to describe chest pain or musculoskeletal pain. This scale is especially useful if you are consulting with a doctor or health professional, as they are generally accustomed to using this scale.

Rating of Claudication (PAD) Discomfort During Exercise Scale

0	No leg discomfort
1	Very, very light
2	Very light
3	
4	Fairly light
5	
6	Somewhat hard
7	
8	Hard
9	Unsteady gait (stop)
10	

If you have peripheral artery disease (PAD), try to exercise as long as possible after onset of pain. Try to tolerate a level of 8 to force muscles to meet their oxygen demand from the available blood supply.

Source: Ciaccia, J.M. *J Vasc. Nursing*, 11: 1-4, 1993.

Appendix E
Learning Pursed Lips Breathing

Pursed Lips Breathing (PLB)

Purpose:

- Helps to keep airways from collapsing during exhale by creating back pressure, making it easier to get "stale" air out
- Reduces rate of breathing and breathlessness

Technique:

- Inhale normally through the nose. If this is not possible, inhale through both the nose and the mouth.
- Exhale through "pursed lips," rounding them as though puckering, or as if whistling. Opening should be as round as possible (can be difficult for some, especially people with dentures).
- Exhale should not be forced; instead let air out passively. If you had a lit candle in front of you, the flame would just flicker rather than be extinguished.
- Exhalation should be at least twice as long as the inhalation (i.e., inhale for two seconds, exhale for four seconds). Exhaling longer may work best for you, and it is fine as long as exhalation is at least twice as long as inhalation.
- Use pursed lips breathing for all physical activity, during times of emotional stress or anxiety, or any time you are short of breath.
- When doing rhythmic activity (walking, vacuuming, mowing lawn), do PLB repetitively. When doing non-repetitive activity, coordinate PLB with movements (i.e., pause as you inhale, and exhale on the effort).

Appendix F
"Finding Muscles I Never Knew I Had"

Note: The body has almost 700 muscles. The following illustrations highlight only the ones that are frequently mentioned in this book.

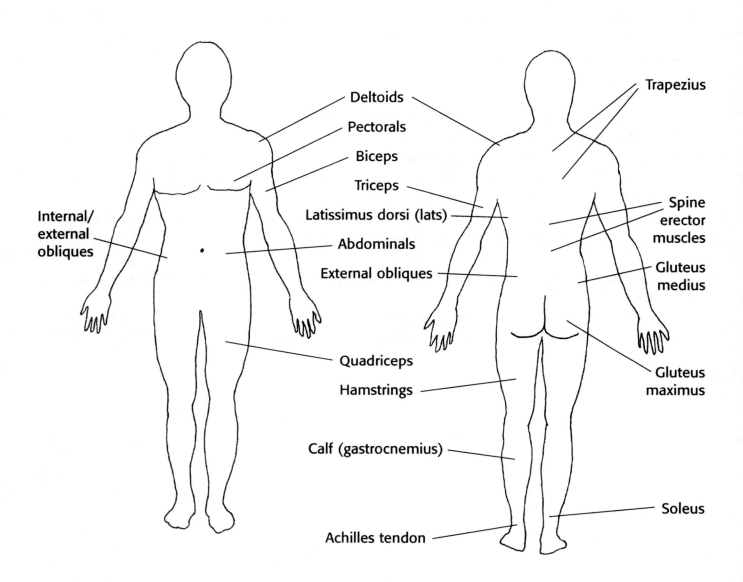

Appendix G
"Making Life A Moving Experience"—Two-Minute Workouts

- *If you can't be more active, be less sedentary:* If working 30 minutes of exercise into your day is a challenge, set a goal instead to subtract 30 minutes of total inactivity.

- *The two-minute workout:* Two-minute blocks of time are relatively easy to find for most people. Incorporate as many two-minute intervals of physical activity throughout your day as possible.

- *Go out of your way:* Make getting there just a little less convenient. Park across the parking lot, park a few blocks away, or get off the bus a few stops early.

- *Go up the down staircase*: Avoid elevators and escalators whenever possible. If you are going up several flights, get off the elevator early and take the stairs the rest of the way.

- *Commercial-robics*: When watching television, use commercial time to get up and move around (this activity may also save you money).

- *Hide-and-don't-seek the remote control:* Do it the old-fashioned way—get up to change the controls (or perhaps get 10-pound remote controls).

- *Break dancing (or walking):* Use your coffee breaks for brisk walking or stretching.

- *Garden with gusto:* Yard and garden chores are effective ways to increase your daily physical activity. It's surprising how many weeds you can pull in two minutes.

- *Clean conditioning:* Use your housework as a way to get more physical activity. Exaggerate reaching, scrubbing and vacuuming motions.

- *Aerobic shopping:* Put on some walking sneakers and do a couple extra laps around the perimeter of the grocery store or mall.

- *Family fitness:* Join your kids and the family dog in physically-oriented activities such as walking, exploring, or outdoor games (this behavior is also important modeling for your children and grandchildren).

- *Activity-to-go:* Make activity convenient when you travel. Stay at a hotel with a fitness facility (and use it), pack walking/running shoes, take walking tours, find community swimming pools or fitness trails, and take your elastic bands with you.

- *No train, no gain:* Delete the adage "No pain, no gain" from your vocabulary. It's consistency that is most important. Stay on track.

Appendix H
The Metabolic Bonfire—How Much Do You Burn at Rest?

Basal Metabolic Rate (BMR) refers to the amount of energy it takes just to keep your vital functions going (i.e., how many calories you burn just to stay alive). All physical activity expenditure is over and above BMR. This figure gives you an idea of how many calories you need to take in (eat) to be in balance (i.e., maintain weight). However, the following factors can also influence this balance.

Men*		Women**	
Weight (lbs.)	Calories/Day	Weight (lbs.)	Calories/Day
140	1,550	100	1,225
160	1,640	120	1,320
180	1,730	140	1,400
200	1,815	160	1,485
220	1,900	180	1,575

*5'10" tall (add 20 calories for each inch taller, subtract 20 calories for each inch shorter)

**5'6" tall (add 20 calories for each inch taller, subtract 20 calories for each inch shorter)

Basal: Minimum amount of energy required (expressed in calories) to sustain the body's vital functions in the waking state.

Factors Affecting Your Basal Metabolic Rate (BMR)

Gender: 5 to 10 percent higher in men than women at all ages.

Body Size: The greater the size (height and weight), the higher the BMR.

Physical Activity: Most profound effect on BMR.

Percentage Body Fat: The higher the percent body fat, the lower the BMR.

Age: The older you are, the lower the BMR.

Amount of Sleep: The more you sleep, the lower the BMR.

Temperature: BMR increases in both hot and cold climates.

Eating (Dietary-induced Thermogenesis): Increases BMR by 10 to 35 percent.

Genetics: Your heredity can greatly influence how effectively your body burns calories.

Appendix I
How Much Does It Cost?—Energy Expenditure of Activities

Approximate Energy Costs in Each 15 Minutes of Various Activities

Physical Activity		*Calories per 15 Minutes (150 lb. individual)*
Aerobic dancing		105
Badminton		99
Ballroom dancing, continuous		53
Basketball		141
Canoeing (recreational)		45
Cleaning house (steady movement)		63
Climbing hills (steady pace)		123
Cooking dinner		47
Cycling	5.5 mph, level ground	66
	9.4 mph, level ground	102
Football		135
Gardening (raking)		56
Golf (walking, no cart)		87
Gymnastics		88
Horseback riding	walking	42
	trotting (English style)	113
Judo		199
Piano playing		41
Rowing machine (fast pace)		105
Running	11 min, 30 sec/mile	138
	10 min/mile	174
	9 min/mile	197
	8 min/mile	213
	7 min/mile	234
	6 min/mile	260
Skiing	cross country, walking pace	146
	downhill	101
Swimming	freestyle, moderate pace	143
	sidestroke	125
Table tennis		69
Tennis		111
Typing (computer)		27
Volleyball		51
Walking	3 mph, level ground	66
	4 mph, level ground	99
	downstairs, steady pace	50
	upstairs, slow steady pace	151
	3.5 mph, ploughed field	108
	3.5 mph, sand dune	130

Appendix J
What Is Your Body Mass Index (BMI)?

Body Mass Index (BMI) at Specific Heights and Weights

Body Weight (lbs.)

Height (in)	19	20	21	22	23	24	25	26	27	28	29	30	31	32	33	34	35	36	37	38	39	40	41	42	43	44	45	46	47	48	49	50	51	52	53	54
58	91	96	100	105	110	115	119	124	129	134	138	143	148	153	158	162	167	172	177	181	186	191	196	201	205	210	215	220	224	229	234	239	244	248	253	258
59	94	99	104	109	114	119	124	128	133	138	143	148	153	158	163	168	173	178	183	188	193	198	203	208	212	217	222	227	232	237	242	247	252	257	262	267
60	97	102	107	112	118	123	128	133	138	143	148	153	158	163	168	174	179	184	189	194	199	204	209	215	220	225	230	235	240	245	250	255	261	266	271	276
61	100	106	111	116	122	127	132	137	143	148	153	158	164	169	174	180	185	190	195	201	206	211	217	222	227	232	238	243	248	254	259	264	269	275	280	285
62	104	109	115	120	126	131	136	142	147	153	158	164	169	175	180	186	191	196	202	207	213	218	224	229	235	240	246	251	256	262	267	273	278	284	289	295
63	107	113	118	124	130	135	141	146	152	158	163	169	175	180	186	191	197	203	208	214	220	225	231	237	242	248	254	259	265	270	278	282	287	293	299	304
64	110	116	122	128	134	140	145	151	157	163	169	174	180	186	192	197	204	209	215	221	227	232	238	244	250	256	262	267	273	279	285	291	296	302	308	314
65	114	120	126	132	138	144	150	156	162	168	174	180	186	192	198	204	210	216	222	228	234	240	246	252	258	264	270	276	282	288	294	300	306	312	318	324
66	118	124	130	136	142	148	155	161	167	173	179	186	192	198	204	210	216	223	229	235	241	247	253	260	266	272	278	284	291	297	303	309	315	322	328	334
67	121	127	134	140	146	153	159	166	172	178	185	191	198	204	211	217	223	230	236	242	249	255	261	268	274	280	287	293	299	306	312	319	325	331	338	344
68	125	131	138	144	151	158	164	171	177	184	190	197	203	210	216	223	230	236	243	249	256	262	269	276	282	289	295	302	308	315	322	328	335	341	348	354
69	128	135	142	149	155	162	169	176	182	189	196	203	209	216	223	230	236	243	250	257	263	270	277	284	291	297	304	311	318	324	331	338	345	351	358	365
70	132	139	146	153	160	167	174	181	188	195	202	209	216	222	229	236	243	250	257	264	271	278	285	292	299	306	313	320	327	334	341	348	355	362	369	376
71	136	143	150	157	165	172	179	186	193	200	208	215	222	229	236	243	250	257	265	272	279	286	293	301	308	315	322	329	338	343	351	358	365	372	379	386
72	140	147	154	162	169	177	184	191	199	206	213	221	228	235	242	250	258	265	272	279	287	294	302	309	316	324	331	338	346	353	361	368	375	383	390	397
73	144	151	159	166	174	182	189	197	204	212	219	227	235	242	250	257	265	272	280	288	295	302	310	318	325	333	340	348	355	363	371	378	386	393	401	408
74	148	155	163	171	179	186	194	202	210	218	225	233	241	249	256	264	272	280	287	295	303	311	319	326	334	342	350	358	365	373	381	389	396	404	412	420
75	152	160	168	176	184	192	200	208	216	224	232	240	248	256	264	272	279	287	295	303	311	319	327	335	343	351	359	367	375	383	391	399	407	415	423	431
76	156	164	172	180	189	197	205	213	221	230	238	246	254	263	271	279	287	295	304	312	320	328	336	344	353	361	369	377	385	394	402	410	418	426	435	443
BMI (kg/m²)	19	20	21	22	23	24	25	26	27	28	29	30	31	32	33	34	35	36	37	38	39	40	41	42	43	44	45	46	47	48	49	50	51	52	53	54
	Normal						Overweight					Obese I					Obese II					Obese III															

BMI calculation for weights outside this chart:

$$\frac{700 \times \text{Weight (lbs.)}}{\text{Height (inches)}^2}$$

Appendix K
Are You Ready?—Stages of Change Model

Adopting a physically active lifestyle is easier for some than for others, and some people are more successful at maintaining it long-term than others. Researchers have identified five stages of change that most people go through as they adopt—or attempt to adopt—new behaviors and habits.

According to this model (Prochaska & DiClemente, 1983), which was initially developed while studying people who quit smoking, the following five specific stages involve both the motivation to change and the actual behavior change.

- Stage One: Precontemplation—You're inactive and "not thinking about it."
- Stage Two: Contemplation—You're inactive and "thinking about it."
- Stage Three: Preparation—You're doing some activity but irregularly.
- Stage Four: Action—You're doing enough activity but have been for 6 months or less.
- Stage Five: Maintenance—Activity is a habit, and you've been doing it six months or longer.

This model is thought of more in a circle, as people will frequently move from one stage into another, and then slide back to an earlier stage. Also, success may not come until many cycles are repeated. It is the well-known concept of "one step forward, two steps back." Behavior change is not easy.

Appendix L
Setting Monthly Goals

> May be copied for ongoing use

Suggestion: Decide what your long-term goal is (i.e., what would you like to achieve by this time next year?). Try to choose a small physical activity goal and a nutrition goal each month that are aligned with achieving your long-term goal. Make the goals realistic. Re-evaluate each month. Notice long-term patterns that are changing over time.

Today's Date _____

Statement of Long-Term Goal (consider 1 year):

_____

Beginning Date _____

_____

Date Achieved _____

_____

Specific Statement of My Monthly Goals (choose one physical activity and one nutrition goal):

1. _____

2. _____

Benefits From Achieving My Monthly Goals:

1. _____

2. _____

3. _____

Possible Obstacles:

How I Will Overcome Obstacles:

_____   _____

_____   _____

_____   _____

_____   _____

Specific Actions I Will Take to Achieve My Monthly Goals:

1. _____

2. _____

3. _____

Positive Affirmations to Help Me Stay on Track:

I recognize the above as a realistic and worthwhile goal. I will approach this goal with positive, constructive energy, and I will achieve success one month from the start date noted on this page.

_____   _____
(Signature)   (Date)